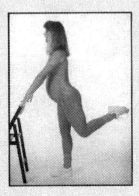

How to Stay Fit and Healthy

Through the Nine Months—

and Shape Up After Baby

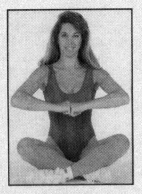

Denise Austin's *Ultimate* Pregnancy Book

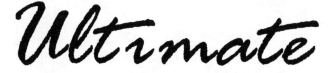

Denise Austin

A FIRESIDE BOOK
PUBLISHED BY SIMON & SCHUSTER

F

FIRESIDE

Rockefeller Center

1230 Avenue of the Americas

New York, NY 10020

FIRESIDE and colophon are registered trademarks

of Simon & Schuster Inc.

Designed by Barbara M. Bachman

Manufactured in the United States of America

1   3   5   7   9   10   8   6   4   2

Library of Congress Cataloging-in-Publication Data

Austin, Denise.

[Ultimate pregnancy book]

Denise Austin's ultimate pregnancy book : how to stay fit and healthy through

the nine months—and shape up after baby / Denise Austin.

p.   cm.

"A Fireside book."

1. Exercise for pregnant women.   2. Pregnant women—Health and hygiene.

3. Pregnancy—Nutritional aspects.   4. Physical fitness for women.   I. Title.

RG558.7.A87   1999

618.2'4—dc21   99-13378

CIP

ISBN 0-684-80219-8

The instructions and advice in this book are in no way intended as a substitute

for medical counseling. We advise the reader to consult with his/her doctor

before beginning this or any regimen of exercise. The author and the publisher

disclaim any liability or loss, personal or otherwise, resulting from the

procedures in this book.

Acknowledgments

I love my girls every minute of the day . . . and I thank God for having two healthy and happy daughters.

I am especially grateful to my husband, Jeff, for all his love and support 100 percent of the time . . . and I love our life together, raising our daughters and sharing this wonderful experience as parents.

Thank you to my cute little mom for having five kids and giving us our big family. I cherish our family's togetherness and it's all because of you.

To my dad who taught us that our positive attitude toward each other and faith in God are both so important.

To my three sisters and my brother . . . we are forever friends. Thank you all for having kids. It is so much fun to see our family tree growing and growing.

Thanks . . . a big thanks to my close friend Stephanie Mansfield for helping me write this book. You are so talented but yet took the time to sit with me for hours laughing and crying about our birth stories and more! For this friendship and support I am ever grateful.

Special thanks to my obstetrician/gynecologist for over fifteen years, Dr. Joseph Giere, for his expertise in the latest medical information on pregnancy and exercise, which he promotes enthusiastically. To Sara Kooperman (Prenatal Exercise Specialist), many thanks for sharing all of your research and knowledge . . . plus working out during all four pregnancies! And to Leslie Bonci, registered dietician and spokesperson for the American Dietetic Association, thank you for your help in planning healthful, nutritious meals.

To my editor, Betsy Radin Herman, and her assistant, Matt Walker, and my literary agent, Jan Miller, thanks for all of your patience, guidance, and encouragement. And to Liza Ashburn, my assistant, thanks for helping me sift through all of my research and organize it into the final project.

I cherish being a mother more than anything, and thanks to all my friends who journeyed into motherhood with me—how we love to share our joys and trials and learn from one another.

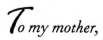

To my mother,

who taught me how to be a loving daughter,

and to my daughters,

who taught me how to be a loving mother

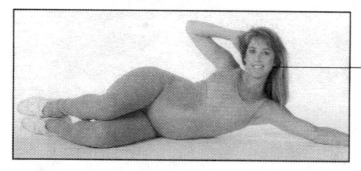

Contents

Introduction

Hi, I'm Denise Austin!

Some of you may know me from my television show, or you may have one of my exercise videos, or you may have seen me on talk shows and in magazines. Well, for the last twenty years I've been coming into your living rooms, encouraging you to get fit, saying, "You can do it!" and "You are worth it!"

And now that you're pregnant, you have the best reason in the world to treat yourself *and* your baby to the greatest gift: the gift of health. Pregnancy is a blessing, and nothing is more important than giving your baby the best start in life. Yes, I've had a successful career, but nothing compares with having a child. I was so thrilled when I first learned I was pregnant, and I knew I was carrying a precious new life. Like you, I worried about how I would stay fit, eat right, give birth, and get back in shape after the baby was born. Don't worry . . . you will!

First of all, I want you to know I'm not a fanatic. I'm not a health nut. I'm not a member of the "fat police." I work hard to have a fulfilling career and to be a loving wife to my husband, Jeff, who is a sports attorney. I'm forty-one now, and we are celebrating our fifteenth wedding anniversary. I'm so luck to have the best husband. I couldn't do what I do without him.

My proudest achievement is having given birth to my two beautiful daughters, Kelly Angela (age eight) and Katherine Reed (age five), whom we call Katie. Nothing has given me more happiness and fulfillment than being a mother, and nothing you will ever do will change your life as much. My life is complete, thanks to my family.

And just like you, I try to maintain an attractive home, although it's far from spotless. I support my community and church and take time out for friends and school volunteering. I drive the girls to gymnastics and tennis just as you do, or will be doing soon. And yes, sometimes I pig out on junk food and skip exercising. Luckily those times don't seem to last too long. I know how much better I look and feel and how much more energy I have if I do work out even if it's only a walk with a girl-friend.

If my day sounds busy, it is. But I always knew I wanted a family, and combining a career and two small children is worth it . . . hectic, but worth it. But the rewards are so great, I wouldn't change a moment of it. I know how much I've been blessed. Truly, my happiest moments are with our little family.

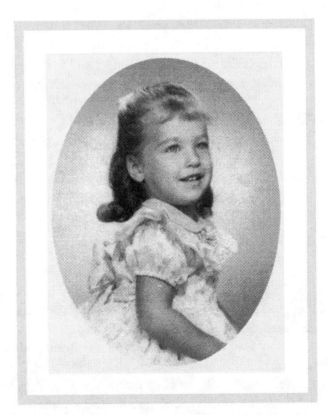

This is me, at age four; my dad's favorite photo of me.

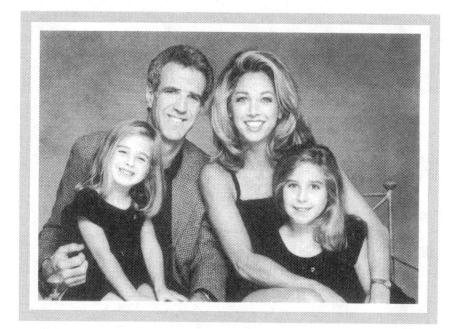

Smile! We're not always this dressed up.

I began thinking about this book while I was pregnant with Kelly eight years ago. I started saving everything I could find on the subject. I interviewed doctors, fitness specialists, and nutritionists and began researching the benefits of exercise during pregnancy. It really was a labor of love! I jotted down sample daily menus for each trimester and gave them to pregnant friends who asked. Having had two successful pregnancies (thank God) doesn't make me an expert in everything, but I have learned a great deal, and now I want to share that knowledge with you.

And yes, as you can see, I gained thirty-five pounds with both babies (and I'm only 5'4")! But I was back in pretty good shape within six weeks. While this is probably due partly to genetics, I attribute this success to my healthy lifestyle. I learned how to modify my exercise programs for each stage of pregnancy and how to bounce back quickly after each birth.

In a way, this book is a natural outgrowth of my two great loves: family and fitness. It is also the culmination of years of hard work.

That's *really* me on the front cover, eight months pregnant. I'm proud that I stayed in shape during both my pregnancies, and I want to teach you how, too!

*E*nter a room with confidence and purpose. No one in the world is exactly like you—you are special in your own way. Especially now that you're about to become a mother.

The pictures you will see in this book are unretouched. For each trimester I wanted a record of my progress. (Yes, there were days I struggled to fit into my leotard.) And my hairstyles look a little out-of-date. But I was determined to keep a true record of each stage of pregnancy. I want you to feel as proud as I did, with each added inch and pound.

This is the most glorious time to be a woman. Yes, there are days you will feel tired and listless. I know I did. You will wonder at the changes in your body. But the time goes so quickly, and believe me, you will always look back on this as the most important period of your life. You are about to give birth. Having a healthy pregnancy is giving your child a head start.

And when you hold your baby for the first time, you will understand. Nothing teaches you more about the true meaning of love. My children mean the whole world to me.

How to Use This Book

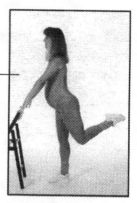

I have divided this book into four sections: the three trimesters of pregnancy and the shape-up after baby.

For each trimester there are three chapters that focus on a healthy and fit pregnancy.

- **HOW TO STAY POSITIVE . . . ALWAYS**
- **HOW TO EAT RIGHT WHILE EXPECTING—AND AFTER!**
- **HOW TO STAY FIT THROUGHOUT YOUR PREGNANCY**

FIRST TRIMESTER:

You will find important nutrition information, diet tips, ways to ease morning sickness, advice on weight gain, and recent health updates. You will also find easy recipes for tummy-soothing meals, as well as an energy-boosting daily exercise routine (always following your doctor's advice) and personal stories of friends and family. And with each section I've included answers to the most commonly asked questions, *plus* a quick and easy sample daily menu for you to follow, which includes all the added vitamins and minerals you will need for a healthy start in these critical first thirteen weeks of pregnancy.

SECOND TRIMESTER:

Now you're feeling energized. Your appetite has returned and you are up, up, up! This is the best time of your pregnancy, fourteen to twenty-nine weeks. I've included quick and delicious recipes, safety tips on continuing your favorite exercise programs, ways to curb food cravings, how to maintain a gradual weight gain, how to avoid stretch marks, and surefire stress relievers.

THIRD TRIMESTER:

You're in the home stretch now, twenty-nine weeks and onward! I've designed specific exercises for that expanding tummy, great stretches for that tired back, soothing circulatory massages. Learn how to choose "good carbs," following my secret plan for snacking "do's and don'ts," know how to get a comfortable night's sleep, and practice my favorite pelvic floor exercises to prepare you for the ultimate experience of childbirth and delivery.

SHAPE UP AFTER BABY:

I will teach you how to bounce back, better than before! We start with postpartum exercises right in the hospital and gradually return to an easy and quick daily routine. Read how to flatten that tummy, lose those extra pounds, eat right (especially if you are nursing), and most important, how to stay well rested, positive, and energized.

Are you ready? Let's *go*.

> *Y*our mind can hold only one thought at a time.
> Make it a positive one.

Part One

First Trimester

CHAPTER 1

"I Can't Believe It. I'm Pregnant!"

All I kept saying was, "I can't believe it. I'm *really* pregnant."

We were going to have our own little baby and become a family. I wanted to tell the whole world. I was so thrilled and excited. I know some people say you're supposed to wait until after the twelfth to thirteenth week, but I couldn't help myself.

I'm from a big Catholic family. My mom and dad had four girls and one boy, and all my sisters and my brother had had children. I knew I always wanted to have kids. Having a family was the most important thing to me. I never wanted to be just a career woman. Jeff is from a big family, too; he's one of five kids. So we couldn't imagine life without building our own family.

There were already lots of grandchildren on both sides, so my family was never pushing me to have a baby. It was usually my friends. I share everything with my sisters, so of course this was a "big topic." Even before I went to the doctor, I called my sisters and told them the pregnancy test was positive. They screamed! They were so happy for us. Since I talk to my sisters almost every day, they got the details of both pregnancies, and I mean *everything*—so let me share it with you!

One of the fears I shared with them was having to get into a leotard for my work. But guess what! Some of my biggest career accomplishments and successes came while I was pregnant. So if you *are* a career woman, don't worry that motherhood will interrupt your career path. It won't. In fact, it will probably make you a more efficient, as well as happier, person. Nurturing a child will bring you the greatest rewards, and love will never seem richer.

If you think you're in love with your husband *now,* just wait until you experience the complete joy of having a child together. It will enrich both your lives and your marriage.

After I took the home pregnancy test, I went to the doctor for a blood test. It was positive. Wow! I'm going to be a mother. Now it was for real. He gave me my due date, which was August 11. I thought to myself, well, that would give me six weeks to get back into shape after delivery because I was scheduled to begin filming my television show on October 1.

Like you, I had hundreds of questions for the doctor; he also had questions for me. He wanted to know about my medical history. I told him everything I knew, and fortunately there was nothing in my family background to suggest I would not have a healthy baby or healthy pregnancy.

My biggest concern was whether I would be able to continue exercising and keep up my travel schedule while filming my television show. Would it be safe to do aerobics? I didn't want to do anything that would harm my baby, and I even told my doctor I would quit my job to have a safe pregnancy. He assured me that I did not have to stop everything. I could continue my regular 30-minute-a-day exercise routine and continue traveling as long as everything was going well.

In fact, research by James F. Clapp, M.D., the world's foremost researcher in the area of exercise and pregnancy, has documented that exercise can reduce labor time by two hours. Exercise during pregnancy can decrease the incidence of C-section by 24 percent, reduce the usage

> One detail researchers now suggest is that obstetricians be aware of whether you were a premie. According to a recent University of Utah study, women born before thirty-seven weeks' gestation have nearly a 20 percent greater chance of delivering prematurely—and the risk more than doubles for women born before thirty-two weeks. Since premature births account for nearly 70 percent of newborn deaths of otherwise normal babies, it's important for your doctor to monitor you. So remember, tell your doctor everything!

of forceps by about 14 percent, and help babies have higher APGAR (responsiveness) scores when born. Dr. Clapp was also recently published in the Journal of Pediatrics documenting that children of women who exercised when they were pregnant had significantly higher general intelligence and better language skills! Exercise is not only healthy for the mother but also important for the child's future.

I continued exercising on a regular basis, and kept up my schedule. The good thing is, I gave up junk food right away and made every calorie count. That's what I can help you do, too.

You—and your baby—are worth it!

Many women say they know they are pregnant almost from the moment they conceive. I didn't know. I even thought I felt menstrual cramps. My period was always "on time," so when I was just one day late I ran out and bought the home pregnancy test. But I still felt a slight bit of cramping those first few days after I knew I was pregnant.

Did you know . . . that cramps signal a change in the uterus? The placenta begins growing before the baby does and is the first functioning organ of the fetus. For the **first three weeks** of pregnancy (before you even realize you have conceived) only the placenta grows—the embryo stays just two or three layers of cells. In addition, some women may even spot a little during this time. This is quite normal.

Fetal growth begins after this stage. Cells in the placenta stimulate production of progesterone from your body, which is needed to maintain the pregnancy.

The placenta is not completely attached, so if you haven't taken the best care of yourself yet, don't worry.

There were other changes.

By **eight weeks** I was having morning sickness that lasted well into the afternoon and evening. On and off, for the next four weeks, the nausea continued. Mostly it was dry heaves; I never actually threw up. I ate so much bread and noodles and carbohydrates just to make me feel better. I felt as though I had a permanent hangover, and the bread would soak up the acid in my stomach. The thought of spaghetti sauce or anything with tomatoes would make me gag. Tomatoes are high in acid and acid made me queasy. I remember not being able to stand the smell of broccoli cooking or hamburger meat. I discovered **ginger** actually helped and ate ginger snaps and put ginger root into my fruit smoothies. **Ginger tea** is also soothing to the stomach.

Antinausea tip . . . To calm a queasy tummy, try a simple fruit dish of chopped crystallized ginger mixed with a teaspoon each of honey and lime juice, mixed with watermelon balls. It's so refreshing and can be stored in an airtight container and snacked on during the day.

I also tried root beer, which one of my friends swore by, and sometimes it helped. *And* it has no caffeine.

Keep crackers everywhere: on your nightstand, in the car, and at work.

Did you know . . . that research now shows that as few as three cups of a caffeinated beverage a day may increase your chances of having a miscarriage and may place the fetus at risk for growth retardation and increased heart rate? Caffeine encourages dehydration, which is a way to lose water-soluble vitamins. Because caffeine is an acid, it promotes calcium secretion in the urine.

I kept eating rice, whole-wheat bread, and plain pasta noodles to feel better, and sometimes it worked. I also gained five pounds, very quickly. Don't be afraid to gain weight. Hormones are stored in body fat.

Fresh air always made me feel better. A walk around the block cleared my head. I often felt nauseated riding in the car. I couldn't sit in the backseat. I had to drive or be in the passenger seat. I would always open up the car window. Jeff would be freezing, and I would say, "But I need fresh air."

Even that winter, I opened the windows of my house every day for several hours to get fresh air.

Dear Denise

I've been eating oatmeal and Raisin Bran cereal for dinner every night for the first three months. I'm afraid I'm not getting enough nutrients for the baby. Help!

Don't worry. If you are concerned enough, ask your doctor. But the baby will get enough nutrients during these first few months without overloading on calories. You don't need to eat a lot more, just one hundred to two hundred calories extra per day, depending on how active you are.

You will need **one hundred more calories if relatively sedentary, two hundred more calories if exercising fifteen to twenty minutes.**

To calm my stomach, I also began eating smaller meals instead of concentrating on three main ones. To keep your blood sugar and energy levels up, try snacking during the day on wholesome foods.

*D*ecide now how you want the rest of your life to turn out. Pregnancy is a time of hope. Believe you can have more than you do, and you will.

FIRST TRIMESTER EATING TIPS

- **KEEP DRY CRACKERS ON YOUR NIGHTSTAND AND EAT A FEW BEFORE YOU GET OUT OF BED IN THE MORNING.**
- **EAT SMALL AMOUNTS OF BLAND FOODS THROUGHOUT THE DAY.**
- **IF IT DOESN'T APPEAL TO YOUR SENSE OF SMELL, IT WON'T APPEAL TO YOUR STOMACH.**
- **TAKE YOUR PRENATAL "HORSE PILL" AT NIGHT OR SPLIT IT AND TAKE HALF WITH BREAKFAST AND HALF WITH DINNER.**
- **TAKE FOLIC ACID.**
- **TRY SUCKING ON A NATURAL LICORICE DROP OR BLACK LICORICE CANDY. IT WILL SOOTHE YOUR STOMACH.**
- **CEREAL IS ALWAYS A GOOD BET, EITHER WITH SKIM MILK OR DRY. CHEERIOS IN A PLASTIC BAG CAN BE A QUICK SNACK. OR A PIECE OF SWEET FRUIT, LIKE A RIPE PEACH, WEDGES OF CANTALOUPE, OR CUBES OF WATERMELON.**

Dear Denise

I haven't had any morning sickness at all. Is there something wrong?

No! My sister Donna felt great in her first trimester and actually worried that her pregnancy wasn't normal. But she just delivered a healthy baby boy and never once felt any morning sickness. (Lucky her!) Remember, every pregnancy is different, and every woman responds differently to hormonal changes in the body.

PREGNANCY IS A time to play it safe, especially in the crucial first few months. Do me a favor and call your doctor if you have *any* questions. It will be a tremendous relief for you and everyone around you. Promise me you will never feel embarrassed: you deserve to know.

Pregnancy is a time of excitement, but also of caution. I get many letters from pregnant women asking if certain things are safe to do, and not just exercise and diet. Remember, ask your doctor if you have any concerns. But there are a few guidelines to follow:

- If you or a family member have exotic pets like lizards, snakes, or other reptiles, check with your doctor about handling them. Many health care providers warn that they carry infections (like salmonella).
- Avoid the use of pesticides and fumigants, and also avoid contact with flea collars and insecticide strips.
- If you must use a spray, wear gloves and keep windows and doors open.
- Avoid oven cleaners and dry-cleaning agents.
- Have someone else in the family change the kitty litter box; cat feces can contain a parasite that causes a rare but serious blood infection, toxoplasmosis.
- Most doctors recommend that you postpone having X-rays of any kind during pregnancy.
- Wash produce before eating.
- Don't exercise outdoors on overly humid or smoggy days.
- If you live in a farm area, or drink from a household well, make sure the water has been tested, especially for pesticides and nitrates.
- Avoid eating shellfish or fish caught in contaminated waters.

FIRST TRIMESTER HEALTH QUESTIONS

Q. *What are the changes I should make in my diet during the first trimester?*
A. *Common sense tells you to give up caffeine, alcohol, and, of course, smoking and drugs. Don't take aspirin or antibiotics without consulting your doctor.*

Here's a way to calculate your due date: Count back three months from the first day of your last period, then add seven days to that number. Or just ask your doctor.

You will need extra calcium, found in milk or skim milk, low-fat cheeses, and low-fat yogurt. Your doctor will likely give you a food chart at your first visit and a prescription for a vitamin supplement.

It's important not to skip meals or starve yourself.

Time is something you can never get back. It's more valuable than money. Focus your time on happy, upbeat, healthy activities. Take time out to spend with friends now, especially ones who are not married or do not have kids. Let them know they are important to you and will be important once the baby arrives.

CHAPTER 2

Eating Smart
for You and Baby

*C*oincidentally, several of my closest friends were also pregnant at the same time. In fact, six of us were pregnant and all due within two or three months of one another. I was one of the last ones, so it was fun to hear what to expect in the upcoming months.

I needed that support group, and it's a good idea now to meet with friends through prenatal classes or groups. Or form your own moms' club . . . it made me feel I wasn't alone.

*T*ake a few minutes each day to relax. It's easy and takes barely any time. Close your eyes, take a few deep breaths, and just let go.

My friends and I enjoyed sharing information about nutrition during these months. Never before has your diet mattered so much; every bite counts!

Some women find it natural to switch to an eating plan high in fresh fruits and vegetables, whole grains, legumes, and low-fat milk products, as well as calcium-rich foods and extra-lean meats. Others who might not have had good eating habits may find it difficult, but now is the time to put aside the sweets and junk food and try to form the *best* eating habits.

Eating enough during pregnancy can help insure a healthy baby, but don't overdo it! Those extra pounds are hard to take off, and the baby needs nutrients, not empty calories. Remember, everything you eat goes to the baby. Your baby needs you to provide all the nutrients necessary to grow properly. What your meals don't give your baby, the baby will take from you. Don't deplete your own energy systems. In the next nine

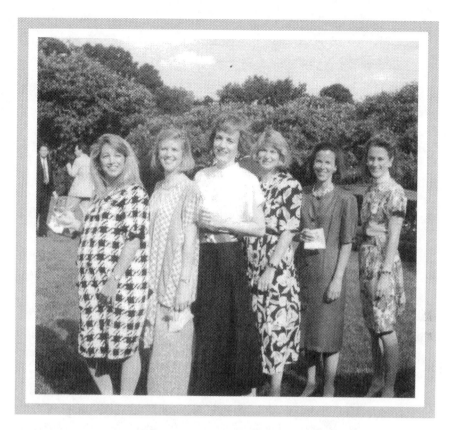

Some of my good friends, all pregnant. I'm the last to go. . . .

months you will be building another human being while keeping your own body healthy.

Your caloric intake needs during the first trimester are virtually the same as they were prepregnancy, and they increase by only one hundred to three hundred calories during the second and third trimesters.

What contains 100 to 300 calories? A flavored yogurt, or an apple and a glass of o.j.

THE AVERAGE WOMAN should expect to gain twenty-four to thirty-five pounds during pregnancy. But don't panic. These pounds are due mostly to the development of the fetus and placenta, the increased amniotic fluid and blood, and expanding uterine and breast tissue. (So, honey, enjoy your new voluptuous figure!)

How *much* you gain is as important as when you gain it. In the first trimester you should aim for a slow, steady gain of two to five pounds. In the last two trimesters your weight should increase by three-quarters to one pound per week. Remember, every woman gains differently. Don't be surprised if you gain six or eight pounds in one week. Just don't do this every week.

And don't forget your prenatal vitamins!

Dear Denise

What's the best time to weigh myself?

Getting on the scale is never pleasant, but now that you're pregnant it's a sign of your baby's growth. The worst time to weigh yourself is after eating a big meal. Also, don't get on the scale immediately after exercising. Fluid loss may make you seem lighter, but only until you drink a few glasses of water.

The best time to weigh yourself is in the morning. Make sure your scale is accurate. Weigh yourself naked, and not more than once a week. Weighing yourself every day is silly, and not an accurate measure of weight gain or loss. I actually kept track of my weight only at the doctor's—I never weighed myself at home.

Most women gain about four pounds in the first trimester.

While your weight may not be going up so much, you will notice subtle changes in the shape of your body, especially your waistline. I certainly did. For someone who always invited you to "feel my tummy," I cut that out of my vocabulary for a while.

If you find yourself quickly gaining more than the recommended amount:

- **AVOID ICE CREAM. DRINK SKIM MILK.**
- **AVOID PASTRIES, CANDY, HIGH-FAT SNACKS. EAT FRESH FRUIT.**
- **BROIL FOOD INSTEAD OF FRYING.**

During the first trimester there are thirteen essential vitamins and minerals that have proved to be beneficial for you and your baby.

Folate, also known as **folic acid**, is crucial for reducing the incidence of neural tube defects in developing babies. The B vitamin is needed to produce the extra blood you and your baby need. Foods high in folic acid are chicken liver, halibut, whole-wheat bread, wheat germ, beets, oranges, Romaine lettuce, spinach, orange juice, and lentils.

Other vitamins like **beta-carotene** assist in the development of the immune system, while **vitamin B_6** is essential in forming all tissues, including the brain, nervous system, and muscles. Here is a chart to help you choose sources of all the vitamins you will need.

Vitamin	Where You'll Find It
Vitamin A	Eggs, liver, dark green or orange veggies
Beta-carotene	Cantaloupe, peaches, sweet potatoes, dark green and orange veggies
Vitamin C	Strawberries, citrus fruits, Brussels sprouts, dark green leafy veggies
Vitamin D	Fortified milk, egg yolk
Vitamin E	Spinach, safflower oil, wheat germ
Vitamin B_2	Asparagus, milk, avocado, salmon, dark green leafy veggies
Niacin	Peanut butter, peas, fish, chicken
Vitamin B_6	Avocado, bananas, potatoes, fish, chicken
Vitamin B_{12}	Eggs, fish, milk, chicken, meat
Biotin	Brown rice, fish, milk, soybeans, peanut butter, oatmeal

Minerals are also found in foods and are crucial for building a healthy baby. **Calcium** builds bones and regulates muscle and nerve function. You will need 1,280 milligrams of calcium daily during your pregnancy. Vegetarians who don't drink milk should consider taking a calcium supplement.

Here are some sample sources of calcium for you and your baby:

8 ounces skim or low-fat milk

1 cup yogurt

1¾ cups low-fat cottage cheese

2 cups broccoli

3 ounces canned sardines

1¾ ounces Swiss cheese

Iron carries oxygen to the baby and to all support tissues, such as the placenta.

Here is a chart to help you insure you get enough minerals in your diet:

Mineral	Where You'll Find It
Calcium	Sardines, dark green leafy vegetables, low-fat milk products, canned salmon
Chromium	Wheat germ, whole grains, orange juice
Copper	Avocado, potato, soybeans, fish, meat, chicken
Iron	Dried apricots, dark green leafy vegetables, raisins, dried beans, potatoes, lean meat
Magnesium	Bananas, peanuts, wheat germ, low-fat milk
Potassium	Fruits, fish, peanuts, veggies
Selenium	Lean meat, seafood, whole grains
Zinc	Wheat germ, dried beans and peas, turkey, lean meat

Water is one of the most important additions to your diet. It is essential for processing nutrients, developing new cells, and sustaining blood volume. Drink six to eight glasses each day; try to carry a bottle of water with you in the car and have one at your desk at work.

Remember: Your urine should be clear. If your urine is yellow, it may mean you are dehydrated. So drink more water!

Unless your doctor has advised otherwise, try to include the following in your new eating plan:

Which Foods?	How Much?	Sample Serving
Dairy	3 servings a day	8 ounces skim milk 1 cup low-fat yogurt 2 ounces cheese ¾ cup cottage cheese
Protein	3 servings a day	2 tablespoons peanut butter 2–3 ounces cooked meat 1 egg ½ cup cooked dried beans
Fruits	3 servings a day	½ cup canned or cooked fruit ½ cup fruit juice 1 medium banana ¼ cup dried fruit
Complex carbohydrates	7–9 servings a day	1 slice whole-grain bread ½ bagel ½ cup cooked pasta, cereal, or rice 1 ounce ready-to-eat cereal
Vegetables	4 servings a day	¾ cup vegetable juice ¾ cup broccoli, carrots, or other vegetables, raw or cooked 1 medium baked potato 1 cup salad

Judge your success not by financial gain, but by the degree to which you are enjoying health, peace, and love. These commodities can never be traded or bartered. Your baby will thank you later.

DENISE'S DIET TIPS

Canned and frozen veggies sometimes can have *more* nutrients than fresh ones. Most prepared vegetables are frozen or processed immediately upon harvesting, while they are at their best. Fresh vegetables continue to lose their nutrients after being picked, and sometimes it takes two weeks for them to get to your market. I prefer fresh vegetables, but if you can't get them or don't want to bother peeling carrots, for example, frozen is great. Watch for the sodium content in canned foods, and stay away from those packed in oils, sauces, syrups, or other additions. Always drain the liquid brine from canned vegetables. You will get rid of 80 percent of the sodium.

Beans . . . are an excellent source of nutrition, and the **cannellini bean** (white bean) has more calcium than any other. **Kidney beans** are a good source of B_6 iron, and **navy beans** are loaded with iron and potassium. **Black-eyed peas** have the most fiber of the group.

Not all lettuce leaves are alike. **Spinach** is by *far* the best salad green you can eat now. It has more nutrients and folic acid than any other type of lettuce. It can also help give you energy. Popeye sure knew his stuff!

One ounce of **Swiss cheese** or four tablespoons of grated **Parmesan cheese** or two cups of **cottage cheese** have as much calcium as an eight-ounce glass of milk. So if you're not a milk lover, there are lots of other sources of calcium.

Pregnancy goes hand in hand with **food cravings,** and more often than not what we are craving is something sweet or high in fat. Make sure fat contributes no more than one-third of your daily calorie count. It's not hard to reduce your fat intake now with all the new products on

Eating well during your pregnancy is an investment in your child's future. Smile! We are baby building!

the market, but beware! Eating an entire bag of fat-free cookies is not the answer. Eating smart *is*.

Pregnancy is a great time to improve the eating habits of your entire family. To know you are eating a well-balanced diet, make sure you get a variety of foods with a reasonable calorie limit, providing all the essential nutrients. Remember: quality, not quantity.

I personally avoided soft drinks, diet drinks, and even herbal teas while I was pregnant. They are all considered "questionable," so why do it? Drink water, skim milk, or fruit juices. Raspberry tea assists with plentiful milk production, eases morning sickness, and helps the uterus stay healthy. *Nettles* tea is high in iron and calcium. It is good for nourishment and helps diminish leg cramps and possibly labor pains. It may also prevent hemorrhoids after birth. Please be careful when using any herbal teas. Some herbs can have stimulating effects, which may bring on early labor.

During my pregnancies, I also found ways to cut down on fat while still enjoying some of my favorite foods.

Here are other ways to reduce your fat intake:

When You Want...	Have...	You'll Save...
A croissant	A whole-grain roll	13 grams of fat
20 French fries	3 boiled new potatoes	16 grams of fat
½ cup shelled peanuts	10 thin pretzels	35 grams of fat
10 potato chips	1 cup air-popped popcorn	7 grams of fat
3 ounces tuna, canned in oil	tuna canned in water	5 grams of fat
1 beef hot dog	turkey hot dog	12 grams of fat
1 slice pecan pie	fruit tart, one crust	23 grams of fat
½ cup ice cream	½ cup frozen yogurt	4 grams of fat

Instead of fried rice, choose steamed rice. Instead of a glazed doughnut, choose an English muffin with jelly. Pour lemon juice over broccoli, not cheddar cheese. Remove the skin from your roasted chicken, and instead of fried fish, switch to broiled fish with lemon juice. Make macaroni and cheese with low-fat sharp cheddar cheese, and replace the milk with evaporated skim milk. For meat loaf, substitute ground turkey.

Note: Research shows that calories from fat go straight into storage in fat cells (most likely your thighs), while calories from carbohydrates are burned for energy.

Eat one gram of fat and you will get nine calories from it. Eat the same amount of a carbohydrate or protein and you'll get only four calories.

ASPARAGUS is a terrific source of B vitamin folate, plus it's virtually fat-free. Eight spears equals 30 calories.

ARTICHOKES are also high in folate, and studies show that women who took extra folate before they conceived had a reduced risk of neural tube defects or congenital malformations in their babies. One medium artichoke equals 55 calories.

BEETS are high in folate and a source of B_2, which helps to energize pregnant women. One cup sliced beets equals 55 calories.

PRUNES AND RAISINS are terrific sources of iron, as well as fiber to help your digestive tract. Five prunes or one-quarter cup raisins equals 115 calories.

MOLASSES is loaded with iron and as a sweetener has other nutritional benefits for mothers-to-be. Two tablespoons of molasses contain nearly as much calcium as a cup of milk. Two tablespoons of molasses equals 85 calories.

PASTA is a terrific complex-carbohydrate food as well as a stress soother. It gives the body energy and also induces calm. But not all pastas are alike. Did you know that the longer the pasta is cooked, the fewer the calories? One cup of pasta cooked to the *al dente* stage is 190 calories. Pasta cooked until tender to the fork is 155 calories.

During my first trimester I did rely on pasta when I couldn't bear the thought of anything else. I learned that not all pastas are alike. Fresh

1 cup white pasta	162 calories	1.5 grams fiber	.8 gram fat
1 cup whole-wheat pasta	174 calories	5.2 grams fiber	.7 gram fat
1 cup spinach pasta	154 calories	1.6 grams fiber	1.2 grams fat
1 cup fresh pasta	149 calories	2 grams fiber	1.2 grams fat

pasta is lower in calories than dried pasta, and whole-wheat pasta is highest in fiber. Spinach pasta is loaded with vitamin A (one cup of cooked spinach pasta has thirty-two grams, compared with white and whole-wheat, which has no vitamin A).

FOOD GUIDE PYRAMID
A Guide to Daily Food Choices

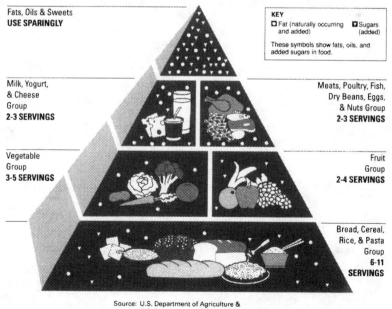

Fats, Oils & Sweets
USE SPARINGLY

KEY
☐ Fat (naturally occurring and added)   ☑ Sugars (added)
These symbols show fats, oils, and added sugars in food.

Milk, Yogurt, & Cheese Group
2-3 SERVINGS

Meats, Poultry, Fish, Dry Beans, Eggs, & Nuts Group
2-3 SERVINGS

Vegetable Group
3-5 SERVINGS

Fruit Group
2-4 SERVINGS

Bread, Cereal, Rice, & Pasta Group
6-11 SERVINGS

Source: U.S. Department of Agriculture &
U.S. Department of Health and Human Services

In the early stages of pregnancy, just keeping food down can be a major challenge! Easy-to-prepare, good-tasting, and small, frequent meals should be the goal, with an extra dose of folate, a B vitamin that plays an extremely important role in your growing baby's health. Calorie needs increase slightly, about 100–300 calories more than you need in a nonpregnant state. Assuming a need for 1,700 calories nonpregnant, pregnancy needs should be roughly 2,000 calories per day.

There are many fad diets out there, recommending high protein and low carbohydrates. There is no benefit in any extremes. During pregnancy, a balanced diet may include 50 percent carbohydrates, 25 percent protein, and 25 percent fat. Don't be scared of pasta. Stick to the food pyramid and enjoy.

MEAL PLANS

Breakfast

¾ cup cereal (flake type or toasted oats) with ¼ cup
  crunch type (low-fat granola)

8 ounces skim milk

2 tablespoons Craisins or raisins

8 ounces orange juice

Midmorning

2 large rice cakes with 1 tablespoon apple butter and
  1 tablespoon peanut butter

8 ounces water

Lunch

1 whole-wheat pita filled with:

3 ounces cubed cooked chicken breast or thigh

½ cup mixed vegetables (frozen or raw)

2 tablespoons "light" dressing

1 tangerine

8 ounces skim milk

Midafternoon

8 ounces decaffeinated or herbal tea

3 gingersnaps

Dinner

1 4-ounce piece white fish baked at 350 degrees, covered
    with sliced onions and spicy stewed tomatoes (fifteen
    minutes to bake)

1½ cups penne pasta (1 cup dry) with 1 tablespoon
    prepared pesto

1 cup steamed broccoli flavored with a splash of soy
    sauce

Juice sparkler: 4 ounces apple juice mixed with
    8 ounces seltzer

Total

Calories: 1,937

Fat: 52 grams

Folate: 295 micrograms

Calcium: 1,229 milligrams

Carbohydrate 53 percent, Protein 23 percent,
    Fat 25 percent

Lentil and Spinach Soup

(Serves 6)

■

This is a delicious first course, packed with vitamin B, protein, and folic acid.

2 TEASPOONS OLIVE OIL
1 ONION, PEELED AND CHOPPED
2 CLOVES GARLIC, MINCED
2 LARGE CARROTS, PEELED AND DICED
2 CUPS DRY LENTILS, RINSED
8 CUPS DEFATTED CHICKEN OR VEAL STOCK
$\frac{1}{2}$ POUND FRESH SPINACH, WASHED AND
ROUGHLY CHOPPED
SALT AND FRESHLY GROUND PEPPER TO TASTE
GARLIC CROUTONS (optional)

Heat olive oil in a Dutch oven or stockpot over low to medium heat. Sauté onions, garlic, and carrots until tender, about five minutes. Add lentils and stock and simmer, partially covered, for twenty minutes. Add spinach and simmer for twenty minutes more until lentils are cooked but not mushy. Season with salt and pepper to taste and serve with toasted garlic croutons if desired.

Pasta and Asparagus in Goat Cheese Sauce

(Serves 4)

■

This is a delicious, tummy-soothing meal. You can also substitute sugar snap peas or thinly sliced zucchini if asparagus is not available.

2 TABLESPOONS BUTTER OR MARGARINE
2 TABLESPOONS ALL-PURPOSE FLOUR
1 CUP DEFATTED CHICKEN BROTH
1 3.5-OUNCE PACKAGE MONTRACHET GOAT
CHEESE, CRUMBLED
1 BUNCH FRESH ASPARAGUS, CUT INTO 2-INCH LENGTHS
OR 1 BOX FROZEN ASPARAGUS *OR*
1 CAN ASPARAGUS, DRAINED OF LIQUID
PINCH OF FRESH OR DRIED ROSEMARY
1 POUND FRESH PASTA (SPINACH, RAVIOLI, OR ANY
MEAT TORTELLINI) OR DRIED LINGUINE
SALT AND PEPPER TO TASTE

Over low to medium heat, melt butter in a medium saucepan. With a whisk or fork, blend in flour and stir. Add chicken broth and heat to boiling, stirring constantly. Turn heat to low and blend in goat cheese until sauce is smooth. Season with salt and pepper, and a pinch of rosemary.

Meanwhile, bring a large pot of water to boil and drop in fresh or frozen asparagus. Cook until tender, about four minutes. (If you are using canned asparagus, simply drain and set aside.)

Remove asparagus from boiling water and set on plate with paper towel to drain. Add pasta to the boiling water and cook according to directions on package.

Drain pasta and toss with asparagus and goat cheese sauce.

Kelly's Quesadilla

(Serves 4)

■

This is an easy version of a Mexican quesadilla, which I love to serve my girlfriends for lunch, with soup, a tossed green salad, and fruit sorbet for dessert. Now my daughter Kelly loves this appetizer, and it's a great way to get her and Katie to eat spinach. Substitute low-fat tortillas and cheese for fewer calories.

$\frac{1}{2}$ 10-OUNCE PACKAGE FROZEN CHOPPED SPINACH,
THAWED AND DRAINED
2 7-INCH REFRIGERATED FLOUR TORTILLAS
$\frac{1}{2}$ CUP SHREDDED MONTEREY JACK CHEESE
2 TABLESPOONS CHOPPED SCALLIONS
$\frac{1}{4}$ CUP SHREDDED WHITE CHEDDAR CHEESE

Heat oven to 450 degrees.

Roll thawed spinach between paper towels to squeeze out the excess water, and chop finely. Place a tortilla on an ungreased baking sheet. Top with the Monterey Jack cheese, scallions, spinach, and cheddar cheese; spread evenly. Place second tortilla on top.

Bake for four minutes. With a spatula, carefully turn over the tortilla and bake four minutes more until cheese has melted and tortillas are crisp.

Cut into quarters and serve with salsa or low-fat sour cream.

Tuna and White Bean Salad

(Serves 4)

■

This is an easy, low-calorie, elegant lunch, loaded with protein. I like to use sweet Vidalia onions, if they are in season, and garnish with black olives and cherry tomatoes.

1 6½-OUNCE CAN WATER-PACKED TUNA, DRAINED
1 14-OUNCE CAN WHITE BEANS, DRAINED
3 TABLESPOONS CHOPPED ONION
½ POUND STEAMED GREEN BEANS, PATTED DRY
4 TABLESPOONS FRESH BASIL, CHOPPED
JUICE OF 1 LEMON
BIBB OR ROMAINE LETTUCE LEAVES

For the dressing:
1 TEASPOON DIJON MUSTARD
2 TEASPOONS RED WINE VINEGAR
1 GARLIC CLOVE, FINELY MINCED
2 TABLESPOONS OLIVE OIL

Place tuna in a mixing bowl, breaking up the chunks with a fork. Toss with the white beans, onion, beans, and basil. Squeeze the juice from the lemon over mixture, and toss lightly. To prepare dressing: In a small bowl, place mustard and add vinegar and garlic. Stir briskly to mix, and add olive oil slowly and steadily in a thin stream. Continue stirring until smooth. Pour over tuna mixture and toss. Serve over lettuce leaves. **This can be made in the morning or afternoon and refrigerated several hours until serving. I still like it best at room temperature.**

Nutrient value: About 208 calories per serving, 20 grams carbohydrate, 6 grams fat, 21 grams protein.

Grilled Salmon with Melon Chutney

(Serves 4)

■

I loved this simple, light fish dish during the first months of my pregnancy. The taste is fabulous, and the cantaloupe gives it extra nutrition. Just one-quarter of a melon supplies as much of vitamins A and C as most people need in one day.

4 SALMON STEAKS
3 TABLESPOONS OLIVE OIL
JUICE OF 1 LIME
1 SMALL MANGO, PEELED AND CHOPPED
½ CANTALOUPE, SLICED INTO QUARTERS
JUICE OF 1 LEMON
1 RED BELL PEPPER, CHOPPED

Place the fish in a bowl or large plastic bag and add olive oil and lime juice. Marinate for a least one hour.

In a food processor, combine rest of ingredients and pulse a few seconds. The chutney should have a chunky rather than mushy consistency.

Grill fish fillets over hot coals until done, about five minutes per side depending on the thickness. Arrange on plate, topped with chutney divided evenly among the four fillets. *Note:* If you don't have a grill, you can bake this fish. Place fillets in glass baking dish, top with the chutney, and bake at 375 degrees until fish flakes easily with a fork, about twenty-five minutes.

Jeff's Favorite Burgers

(Serves 4)

■

Jeff and I were both born and raised in California, and we love to grill. Over the years we have found great ways to enjoy burgers, but without all the fat and calories. You can experiment with the choice of ground meats. Sometimes I use half lean ground beef with ground veal or ground turkey. I've found that mixing the turkey with another meat gives it more flavor and produces a juicier burger.

$\frac{1}{2}$ POUND LEAN GROUND TURKEY
$\frac{1}{2}$ POUND LEAN GROUND BEEF OR LAMB
$\frac{1}{4}$ CUP MEDIUM-HOT SALSA
1 TEASPOON CHILI POWDER
$\frac{1}{4}$ TEASPOON GROUND CUMIN
4 HAMBURGER ROLLS
LETTUCE AND TOMATO SLICES FOR GARNISH

For the garnish:
2 TOMATOES, PEELED, SEEDED, AND CHOPPED
1 AVOCADO, PEELED AND CHOPPED
$\frac{1}{4}$ CUP NONFAT OR LOW-FAT SOUR CREAM
1 TABLESPOON MINCED CILANTRO

Stir together the tomatoes, avocado, sour cream, and cilantro. Set aside.

In a mixing bowl, combine the meats, salsa, chili powder, and ground cumin. Blend well, using your hands, and form into 4 patties. On a well-oiled grill, cook burgers until done. We usually like them about five minutes on each side.

To assemble, place rolls on each plate and divide the tomato-avocado mixture evenly on the bottom of each roll. Place the hamburger on top, garnish with lettuce and slice of tomato.

Denise's Guilt-free Shakes

(Serves 2)

■

**Even my husband enjoyed drinking these
low-calorie "milk" shakes with me during my
first months of pregnancy. They're a
great calcium boost!**

¾ CUP SKIM MILK
½ CUP NONFAT OR LOW-FAT VANILLA YOGURT
1 TEASPOON VANILLA

Place all ingredients in a blender and process until smooth. Serve cold.

Chocolate shake: Add 1 tablespoon Ovaltine.

Strawberry shake: Substitute strawberry yogurt for vanilla, and add 1 cup sliced and hulled fresh strawberries.

Banana shake: Add 1 cup sliced banana, and substitute strawberry-banana yogurt for vanilla.

FIRST TRIMESTER NUTRITION QUESTIONS

Q. *I seem to be tired all the time. Is this normal?*

A. *Yes, especially in the first trimester. For the first few weeks, every afternoon my head would plop down on the desk. I had to fight to keep my eyes open. If you can, lie down and take a ten-minute nap.*

This is a hard time to ask the boss to install a sleep sofa next to your desk, since no one knows you're pregnant. The most important thing is for you to get the most rest you can. That means go to bed early. I was in bed every night by nine P.M. during my first trimester. Make rest your priority!

Q. *Since folic acid is so important for pregnant women, which is the best source—fortified foods or a supplement?*

A. *Recent studies have found that folic acid in six of nine prenatal supplements did not dissolve, which means neither the pregnant woman nor her baby received any nutrient. For that reason I recommend fortified foods such as cereal and pasta as the primary source of folic acid. You will* need 400 micrograms daily, and that means cereal for breakfast, two slices of whole-wheat bread at lunch, 1½ cups of cooked pasta and a roll at dinner. Ask your doctor if you are considering supplements, but I never found it difficult to fit these nutrients into my daily diet. In fact, I still do!

Food isn't the enemy. Sitting still is.

CHAPTER 3

You Can Do It!
Exercises for the
First Trimester

Dear Denise,

I have just found out I am pregnant. Is it still safe to exercise?

Yes! If you have a normal pregnancy and your doctor has approved, not only is it safe to exercise now, it's important for your body to stay active and energized. I continued to work out, mainly doing low-impact aerobics, walking, and lifting light weights to help me feel better. And it did. But I didn't change my work schedule. I continued full steam ahead, filming my show, traveling, making personal appearances, and appearing as a guest on television shows *(Donahue, Good Morning America).*

*W*hen you get down, remember that you are giving the gift of life. It is the most precious gift you will ever give to anyone.

Each week I receive hundreds of letters from women asking for advice. Pregnant women always want to know the same things: Will my hips spread? Will I feel *this* tired for the entire nine months? I can understand how they feel. During those first weeks of pregnancy I remember feeling listless and so tired sometimes, especially after dinner. I remember saying to Jeff, "I just want to feel like my old energetic self again."

There were more questions from expecting moms: Can I still exercise now that I'm pregnant, and how much can I do? What is safe? These are all typical questions. The first and most important thing you must do before beginning any exercise is to consult your doctor. As long as you have a normal pregnancy, you can continue your exercise routine with some modifications.

Think positive thoughts once every hour, and try to envision what your baby looks like at this stage.

The following new American College of Obstetricians and Gynecologists (ACOG) guideliness should be followed by pregnant women:

1. Regular exercise 3 times a week is preferrable to infrequent exercise.
2. Do not lie on your back to exercise after the first trimester.
3. Stop or reduce your exercise level if you get fatigued. Do not exercise to exhaustion.
4. Because of changes in the body, and a reduction in the ability to balance, avoid exercise programs in which falling or other trauma is possible.
5. Be sure to eat enough to accommodate the calories expended in exercise.
6. During the first trimester, be careful to avoid overheating, drink plenty of fluids, wear layered cotton clothes that breathe, and avoid extreme humidity and heat when exercising.
7. Return to exercise gradually, based on your own capabilities.

CONDITIONS THAT RESTRICT EXERCISE

- **PREGNANCY-INDUCED HYPERTENSION**
- **INCOMPETENT CERVIX**
- **PERSISTENT SECOND OR THIRD TRIMESTER BLEEDING**
- **PREMATURE LABOR DURING A PRIOR OR CURRENT PREGNANCY**
- **VAGINAL BLEEDING OR RUPTURED MEMBRANES**
- **INTRAUTERINE GROWTH RETARDATION**
- **CHRONIC HYPERTENSION; OVERACTIVE THYROID; CARDIAC, VASCULAR, OR PULMONARY DISEASE**

- **SUSPECTED FETAL DISTRESS (AS SHOWN THROUGH A SONOGRAM, REDUCED FETAL MOVEMENTS, OR FETAL MONITORING)**

WARNING SIGNS TO STOP EXERCISING

- **VAGINAL BLEEDING**
- **ABDOMINAL OR CHEST PAIN**
- **LEAKING OR GUSHING FROM VAGINA**
- **SUDDEN SWELLING OF HANDS, FACE, OR FEET**
- **SEVERE, PERSISTENT HEADACHES**
- **DIZZINESS OR LIGHT-HEADEDNESS**
- **NOTICEABLE REDUCTION IN FETAL ACTIVITY WHEN NOT EXERCISING**
- **PAINFUL, REDDENED AREA ON THE LEG**
- **SEVERE PAIN IN PUBIC AREA OR HIPS**
- **PAIN OR BURNING SENSATION WHEN URINATING**
- **IRRITATING VAGINAL DISCHARGE**
- **ORAL TEMPERATURE OVER 100 DEGREES**
- **PERSISTENT VOMITING**
- **UTERINE CONTRACTIONS**
- **HEART PALPITATIONS**
- **SHORTNESS OF BREATH**

Since I've exercised most of my life, I was able to continue my fitness routines thoughout both pregnancies. This is what I did: three days a week I continued doing aerobic activities, modifying the intensity slightly. I took it down a notch and tried not to push myself. On Mondays I walked for 30–40 minutes, on Wednesdays I rode a stationary bike and on Fridays I did step aerobics, the step machine, or I would swim for 30 minutes. There are so many ways to get aerobic benefits. The goal is to keep up your favorite form of exercise—with your doctor's approval.

One of the things I did do differently when I was pregnant was to check my heart rate frequently. The best way to make sure that you are not overdoing it is to do a "talk test." If you can talk comfortably, you are exercising at a reasonable level.

On Tuesdays and Thursdays I continued my toning routines, which begin on page 49. These are terrific ways to boost your energy, increase circulation, and tone and firm your muscles.

I always finished up with a few of my favorite stretches, found on page 59.

During my first pregnancy I experienced some vaginal bleeding in the first trimester. I was worried, so I called my doctor. He told me to rest for several days and then resume my fitness routine when I stopped spotting. It is very important to remember that you *cannot* exercise a baby out of you. Absolutely no research has shown that exercise in any form causes miscarriage. If you became pregnant while you were on a fitness program, of course you can continue safely. It is now recommended that if you did not exercise before you became pregnant, now is a great time to begin!

*A*t bedtime, sing a lullaby to your baby. It will help you and your baby relax into a peaceful sleep.

I remember when I heard my first child's heart beat, at **ten weeks**. Jeff came with me to the doctor's office. It was the first time I truly realized a little human being was inside me. Jeff and I both cried with happiness. The baby was only the size of a thumbnail, but what a miracle!

Twelve weeks was the turning point in my pregnancy.

The nausea had subsided. I had my energy back, yes! Finally. I didn't need those afternoon snoozes anymore.

I loved my cup of coffee in the morning, but I had already switched to decaf when I learned I was pregnant. Out went the colas and diet colas. I drank diluted fruit juices, and of course lots of water. Eight glasses a day, throughout my whole pregnancy. The number one thing to remember now and throughout your pregnancy is to keep **hydrated**.

By now I had learned to wear clothes during exercise that didn't inhibit movement; a unitard with a T-shirt, with loose shorts or sweatpants. I found bike shorts and tights uncomfortable as my stomach grew.

*K*eep a journal of your pregnancy. Years later you and your child will treasure it and laugh about your adventure. My daughters love to hear stories of when I was pregnant with them and consider themselves as having experienced the same wonderful things. They even say they met the same people I did, even if they were in my tummy!

You probably will have moved up a bra size. Have you noticed your nipples might be appearing more brown? Mine did. And how about those blue spidery veins that have suddenly appeared on your breasts? I did experience a certain amount of tenderness there, but a good supportive bra helped.

Many women find that wearing a supportive bra while sleeping helps reduce pain. Heat actually increases swelling and may increase discomfort. Reducing your salt intake prevents water retention. Caffeine can also be the culprit; some studies have shown that women who cut caffeine from their diet for one to six months have a 65 percent reduction in breast pain—another reason to switch to decaf!

Warning: Women who use health food remedies have reported that **evening primrose oil** helps reduce breast pain. I don't recommend this treatment for pregnant women, as studies show evening primrose oil has been known to contribute to miscarriages.

Most women experience breast pain, known as **mastaglia,** at some point in their lives. Breast pain is most common during times of hormonal inbalance, such as teenage years and pregnancy.

Breast pain is *not* a sign of cancer. In fact, only 10 percent of breast cancers do cause pain. Fluid retention can cause pain. Chest pain may also be caused by some forms of strength training, such as running with hand weights or bench presses. I don't advise you to run or walk with any sort of hand weights or ankle weights while you're pregnant. (Don't we already weigh enough?) A word of caution (it's just common sense): If anything hurts, stop doing it. As with any exercise, your body will tell you when to slow down. See your doctor if you have any of these symptoms:

- **THE PRESENCE OF A FIRM, UNMOVABLE LUMP**
- **ANY NEW OR UNUSUAL LUMP**
- **THICKENED AND/OR DIMPLED SKIN**
- **A SCALY OR TENDER NIPPLE**
- **NIPPLE DISCHARGE**

Dear Denise

I'm 2½ months pregnant, and I don't seem to have the energy to exercise anymore. Help!

Feel like a wet dishrag? Need motivation to get off the couch and into the gym? Take your husband or partner! It's hard for men to understand the changes your body is undergoing. Sure, we involve them at the end by asking them to take childbirth classes, but now is the best time to share your new healthy regimen. If he's going to eat the same well-balanced meals, exercise with him, too: you are more likely to stick to your workout that way than if you exercise alone. So make a date—to exercise! Afterward share a foot message and enjoy a moment of relaxation.

> *D*o whatever it takes to ensure a healthy baby. Do everything you can to eat right and avoid stressful situations and negative people. Think positive thoughts!

If you don't belong to a gym, take a walk together or go for a swim. I remember Jeff and I used to take long walks together when I was pregnant. Or take your children! While I was pregnant with my second child, Katie, I would put Kelly in the stroller for our walks together. It was fun, and I still treasure those times we shared together.

My husband is a former professional tennis player. His mother, Jeanne, my mother-in-law, played tennis throughout her pregnancy (even back then!) and won a tournament the day she delivered future U.S. Open champion Tracy Austin.

So Tracy began training in her mom's tummy!

TEN MINUTE FIRST TRIMESTER TONING ROUTINE

Exercise is a natural tranquilizer, easing tension and anxiety. You will feel more relaxed, which is beneficial to you and your baby. The benefits of aerobic exercise include:

- **IMPROVED CIRCULATION**
- **ENHANCED BALANCE**
- **REDUCED SWELLING**
- **IMPROVED DIGESTION AND REDUCED CONSTIPATION**
- **FEWER LEG CRAMPS**
- **FASTER POSTPARTUM RECOVERY**
- **FEWER PROBLEMS SUCH AS VARICOSE VEINS, HEMORRHOIDS, BACKACHES, AND MUSCLE OR JOINT SORENESS**
- **INCREASED ENDURANCE**

- **SHORTER LABOR TIME**
- **FEWER C-SECTIONS**
- **LESS USAGE OF FORCEPS**
- **STRONGER MUSCLES MOST AFFECTED BY PREGNANCY: PELVIC FLOOR, ABDOMINALS, AND LOWER BACK**
- **IMPROVED BODY IMAGE, MOOD, AND SENSE OF WELL-BEING**
- **INCREASED METABOLISM, BETTER WEIGHT-GAIN CONTROL**
- **INCREASED STRENGTH AND FLEXIBILITY OF TENDONS AND LIGAMENTS**
- **IMPROVED COORDINATION**
- **IMPROVED EXERCISE AND LABOR TOLERANCE**

Exercising should not be a chore. It should become second nature to you—like brushing your teeth. My goal is for you to do this ten-minute routine, at least four days a week. I did it almost every day, and it helped keep me toned, firm, and feeling energized. It's a great total fitness plan, and you should make it your daily routine. Get into the habit. It can be done in the morning or evening. Try it with your husband!

Don't overdo anything. If something feels as though it might be too much for you to accomplish, don't do it. Save your strength for the most important person in your life: your baby.

Warm-up

∎

Stand with your legs apart, one knee bent. Raise your left arm over your head and release. Then raise your right arm over your head and release. Alternate arms, lunging slowly, using your thigh muscles. Inhale deeply and exhale.

REPEAT 20 times.

BENEFITS: Strengthens thigh muscles and warms up the body for the exercise routine. Elongates the spine for a great stretch. Increases flexibility in arms, shoulders, and lateral trunk muscles.

TRAINER TIP . . . Don't bend over so far that your back is out of line. The key is to lift and elongate.

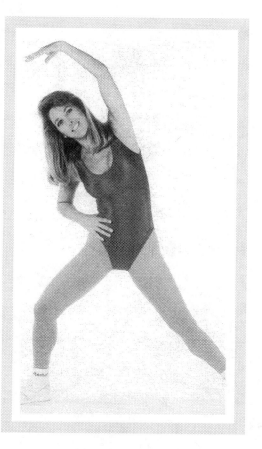

Thigh Toner

Stand with your legs apart, one knee bent, and stretch out your arms as far as they will go. Elongate your body and think "good posture." Rock from side to side, bending your knees slightly. Your knee and ankle should be in a straight line. Try not to let your knee go past your toes. Don't lock your body. Everything is soft.

REPEAT 20 times.

BENEFITS: Strengthens inner thighs, hamstrings, and quadriceps and continues to warm up and tone the body.

Also, this exercise helps with flexibility of pelvis area, which is important during pregnancy.

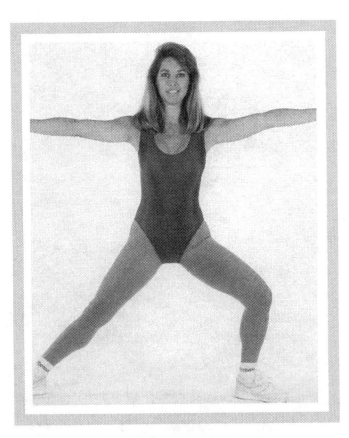

Outer Thigh Trimmer

This is where I gained my extra weight during my first pregnancy. Doing this exercise really helped during my second pregnancy, and I was able to slim down my saddlebags. Watch out for that big tushy! Your weight will settle there unless you continue this exercise.

Stand with your feet together, your hands on the back of a chair for balance. Your back should be straight and your abs tight. With your foot flexed, slowly lift your right leg out to your side, then lower the leg. Be sure to keep your back straight, chest open, and tummy tight. The movement should be slow and deliberate. Repeat. When you have finished your two sets with the right leg, repeat the exercise on the left leg.

REPEAT 2 sets of 8–12 leg lifts each.

BENEFITS: Outer thigh (abductors).

TRAINER TIP . . . When using a chair, make sure it is a sturdy one, without rollers. Try the sofa or a good strong armchair.

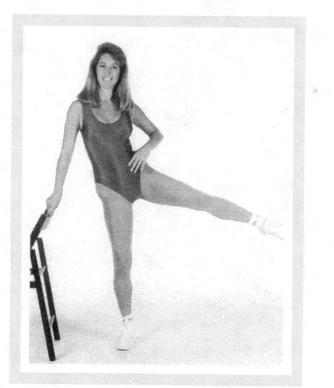

Bun Firmer

Stand with your feet together, your hands on the back of a chair for balance. Your back should be straight and your abs tight. Keeping your hips square to the chair and your right foot flexed, raise your right leg behind you. Keep the right leg straight. As you complete the movement, be sure that you don't arch your back at all; do really squeeze your buttocks.

Return your leg to the starting position and repeat. When you have finished the reps with the right leg, repeat the exercise with the left leg.

REPEAT 2 sets of 8–12 leg lifts each.

BENEFITS: Buttocks (gluteals).

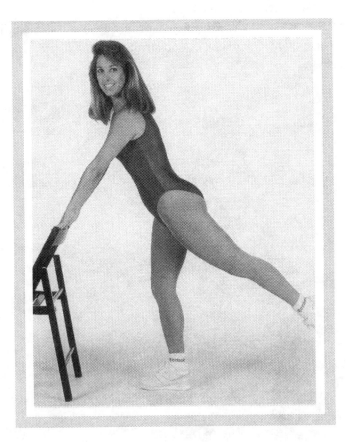

The Pelvic Rock

•

This is an easy exercise that will do wonders for the buns. Make sure you squeeze the buttocks, as if you are squeezing the last drop of water out of a towel. A great bun burner!

Lie on your back, bend your knees, and keep your feet flat on the floor. Extend your arms along your sides. Lift your buttocks off the floor (3–6 inches) by tilting your pelvis up, squeezing your buttocks, and tightening your abs. Hold for a few seconds and slowly rock your left hip slightly. Rock side to side, tilting your pelvis. The movement is diagonal. Hold for a few seconds and lower your bottom down, one vertebrae at a time. Remember that in the fourth month of pregnancy, all back-lying positions will need to be changed. See p. 97 for modifications.

REPEAT 8–12 times, then rest between reps.

BENEFITS: This helps strengthen the pelvic floor muscles, which are important during your pregnancy.

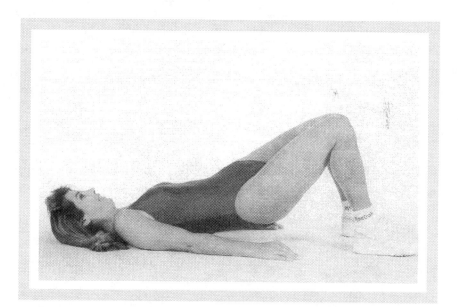

Abdominal Strengthener

This is a great exercise to do during the first trimester, since we can still lie on our backs. After sixteen weeks we must do any ab exercises lying on our sides or standing up. So take advantage now!

Lie on your back with your knees bent and your feet on the floor. (If you are a beginner, or have neck problems, use a pillow under your neck and head.) Press your lower back firmly into the floor. Try to minimize the arch in your back. Rest your head in your hands, but keep your neck and shoulders relaxed. Tighten your abdominals and slowly lift your shoulders up off the floor (about 6 inches). Exhale as you crunch!

Keep your elbows back and your chin up as if you have an apple between your chin and chest. Slowly lower your shoulders back to the floor and repeat.

REPEAT 2 sets of 8–12 crunches each. Rest 15 seconds between sets.

BENEFITS: Abdominals (rectus abdominis).

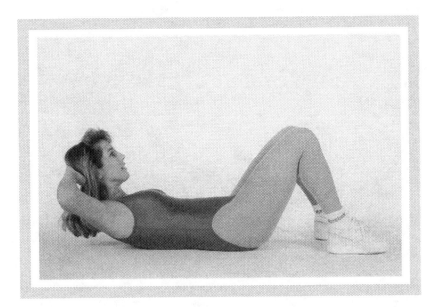

Torso Strengthener

■

Even though you're pregnant, you can still keep "somewhat" of a waist-line by keeping your sides trimmed and toned. Fight those love handles!

Lie on the floor with your knees bent and feet flat.

Press your back firmly onto the floor. There should be little or no arch in your back. Place your right hand out to your side and your left hand behind your head. Exhale as you lift your left shoulder blade off the floor. You are not going to touch your elbow to your opposite knee—just move in that direction. Slowly lower your back to the floor and repeat.

REPEAT 2 sets of 8–12 reps each per side. Rest 15 seconds between sets.

BENEFITS: Waistline (obliques). Helps keep entire area strong and healthy, to prepare you for carrying the baby. Strengthening of your ab muscles will also help your posture, prevent lower back pain, and help you return to your prepregnancy size sooner.

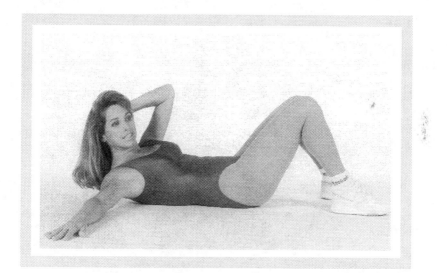

Chest Firmer

Although our breast tissue is mostly fat, exercise can keep the underlying muscles strong and ward off droop, even during pregnancy. Fight gravity with this uplifting routine.

Sit down cross-legged, with your back straight. Press your knuckles against one another. This is an isometric exercise, pressing and pushing and strengthening your upper body. Feel your chest muscles working.

REPEAT each sequence 3 times. Relax for 5 seconds.

BENEFITS: Firms and tones your pecs and arms. Pregnant women often experience soreness in their breasts. This is a good way to strengthen those muscles.

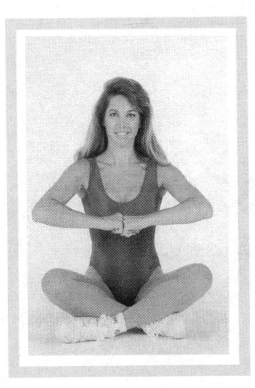

Posture Stretch

Because of weight gain and our changing center of gravity, pregnancy can often result in slouching. Here's a great stretch to open the chest and improve your posture. Slouching can cause neck and shoulder pain and even reduce your energy level.

Sit on the floor, cross-legged. Place your hands behind your head and open up your chest. Feel that wonderful stretch in your upper body. Take a deep breath. Hold for 5 seconds and release.

REPEAT 3 times.

BENEFITS: Improves posture, strengthens upper back muscles. Tones upper back muscles you'll need throughout pregnancy. This exercise also opens the chest and helps the rib cage to expand to accommodate the growing fetus.

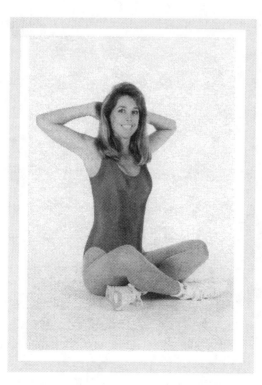

Leg and Back Stretch

I do this stretch all the time, whether I'm in bed, lying on the floor playing with the girls, or just watching television. This is especially useful if your lower back is bothering you (and this can be chronic during pregnancy). Remember to breathe and relax and never bounce. Also, take advantage of this exercise now in your first trimester. You won't be able to continue to exercise on your back after the sixteenth week.

Lie on your back on the floor, with your knees bent and your feet on the floor. Raise your right leg up and pull it toward your chest. You can use a towel to assist you. Hold the stretch for 15–20 seconds. Lower the leg and repeat the stretch with the left leg. To feel the stretch more in your calf muscle, wrap the towel around the ball of your foot.

REPEAT 2 times.

BENEFITS: Terrific exercise for leg (hamstring) cramps, and also promotes circulation.

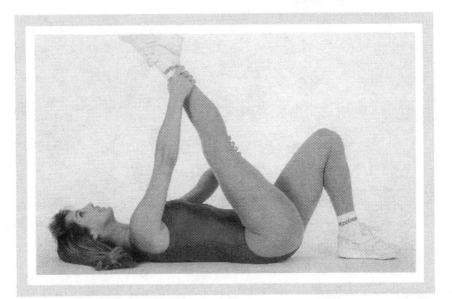

STAYING IN SHAPE during pregnancy does not mean giving up your favorite sport. But it *does* require some modification. Doctors warn us to avoid a sport with a risk of falling, causing abdominal trauma, or quick, sharp changes of direction. You may not have the same balance and coordination, thanks to your enlarged uterus and breasts. And be sure to drink plenty of fluids to avoid dehydration. Keeping properly hydrated helps to avoid cramping. *Tip:* Drink eight ounces before you exercise and eight ounces after.

At about **sixteen weeks** your uterus begins to extend beyond the pelvic bone, making you more vulnerable to injury. During my first pregnancy I didn't "show" until my fourth month. But during my second pregnancy my tummy popped out right away. It seemed as though I showed by six to eight weeks. There's a reason: they call it *muscle memory.* It's the same reason pro golfers can repeat their swings again and again. Your muscles have an unbelievable memory and know what they are supposed to do. I've also heard that like a balloon, once the uterus expands it is stretched and will blow up more easily the second, third, or fourth time around.

*K*eep a pad and pencil by your bed. When you think of a question for your doctor, jot it down and bring it to your next appointment.

As long as your pregnancy is progressing normally, there is no reason to avoid any exercise you enjoy with some minor changes. But it's just common sense that you should not be rock climbing, scuba diving, water skiing, or bungee jumping! Still, there are plenty of other sports for the athletically inclined.

*P*ay attention to your environment. Buy yourself a bunch of tulips or one perfect rose. Play soothing music. It won't be hard to remain serene in that setting.

With a little moderation you can still pursue your favorite activities. As with any exercise program, check with your doctor first. But here are a few guidelines to help maintain the cardiovascular benefits of your sport while taking it down a notch or two:

If your favorite activity is . . .	Switch to
Aerobics, dance	Low impact, and avoid quick changes in direction
Aerobics, step	Lower step 4–6 inches. Avoid jumps and leaps. Be careful. If you look down and can no longer see the step, switch to low-impact aerobics.
Biking	Shorter easier straight rides. Stop if you feel your balance is not right.
Biking (stationary)	A recumbent bike might be better for your back, but any stationary bike is good.
Golf	Nine holes instead of eighteen. Stop if there is back pain. I recommend walking, but if you can, use a caddie. Do not carry your own bag. Or better yet, take a cart. Drink plenty of fluids.
Rollerblading	Walking. Put the skates away.
Skiing	Cross-country only. Stick to easy courses, with few or no hills. Don't ski above ten thousand feet. High altitude can deprive you and the baby of oxygen.
Swimming	Avoid jerky kicks and movements. Stop if your back hurts.
Tennis	Doubles. Avoid jerky, quick stops and starts. Drink plenty of fluids.
Yoga	After the fourth month do not lie on your back. Avoid extreme twists, extreme stretches and back bends.

> *A*ct like an athlete in training. You have
> nine months until your "big event."

Now is the time to get my *Pregnancy Plus* video. It's been a best-seller for years, and I can't tell you how many women write to tell me how it worked for them.

Here's one letter, from a woman in Harrisburg, Pennsylvania, who writes:

Dear Denise,

My pregnancy was a piece of cake thanks to your pregnancy tape. I did it three days a week, and felt great. I gained 40 pounds but lost it all after three months . . . I loved your after-baby shape-ups!"

During the early part of your pregnancy, hormonal surges can cause mood swings, almost like PMS. Just remember, everyone experiences this. Every time I heard a sentimental song about love, family, or babies I became weepy, and sometimes I just bawled. I was crying at every movie, even silly things on television. Every emotion was triggered.

Beauty Tip

During both of my pregnancies my face became fuller. So I made sure I always wore a little makeup to look and feel better. I took an extra minute to pay attention to my eyes. They became the focus of my face, not my chubby cheeks. During the day I highlighted my eyes with a thin liner on top with a brown eyeshadow and mascara. I paid special attention to my eyebrows. Remember, they frame your face. Keep them neat and natural and filled in with brow pencil if needed.

Q. *I just found out I'm pregnant. Can I still do aerobics?*

A. *Yes, you can maintain your normal aerobics classes or videos, as long as you get your doctor's approval. As your pregnancy progresses, you will need to modify your workouts. Remember to stay cool while exercising, drink plenty of water, and wear a supportive bra, supportive shoes, and loose, cool clothing. And most important, can you talk while you exercise without gasping for air?*

Q. *Can I continue weight training throughout my pregnancy?*

A. *Yes, you can, if you have a normal pregnancy. Strong muscle tone is key to staying fit and having the strength to be able to carry the baby until the ninth month (and after!). As your pregnancy progresses, you may notice you are not as comfortable, owing to pressure in the pelvic area or hemorrhoids. Heavy weights are not recommended. However, you can continue to weight train, performing 8–12 reps of an exercise. Make sure you can perform these 8–12 reps without undue strain. It is important to weight-train to help you through the pregnancy and after. You will soon be carrying around your baby without your tummy's help! If you want, lower the weight if this makes you feel comfortable.*

Rest often between reps, and don't hurry. Avoid jerky movements. Keep them slow and steady and smooth. Remember to give yourself 48 hours between weight-training sessions on the same muscle group.

Q. *What about stretching? Is that safe?*

A. *It is safe to continue stretching as long as you take a few precautions. Your hormones are surging, and one of them, relaxin, is making every ligament and tendon more flexible in preparation for childbirth. So stretch in moderation. Never go past your normal point of stretching. Don't be too ambitious. Stretch for release of tension and anxiety. Some women continue to do yoga throughout their pregnancies. Again, ask your doctor before beginning any exercise program. I personally like to stretch after a workout, when my muscles are warm and prepared.*

Don't forget that your husband is about to become a father. He is feeling all sorts of different emotions. Talk to him about his expectations and fears. Now is the time to reassure each other.

Easy-does-it stretches for moms-to-be: Now is a good time to make it a healthy habit to stretch a few minutes every day. Here are my favorite ones I did while expecting . . . and still do.

Quad Stretch

Stand, with one hand holding a chair, a wall, or a friend for balance. Lift one leg behind you, holding your foot and gently pulling your heel toward your buttocks. Feel the stretch in front of your thighs. Hold for 20–30 seconds.

REPEAT 2 times for each leg.

BENEFITS: Stretches front thigh (quadricep) muscles.

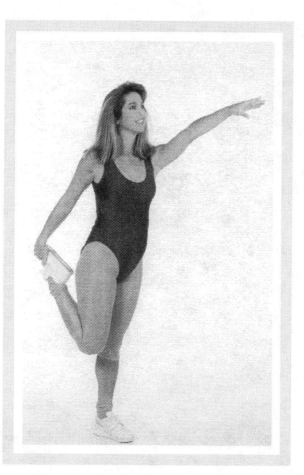

Shoulder Stretch

Put your right hand on your left shoulder. Cup your right elbow with the palm of your left hand. Pull the elbow gently toward your left shoulder. Hold the stretch for 15 seconds, then release. Switch sides and pull your left elbow toward your right shoulder. Repeat.

REPEAT 2 sets with each arm.

BENEFITS: Stretches and relaxes the shoulder muscles.

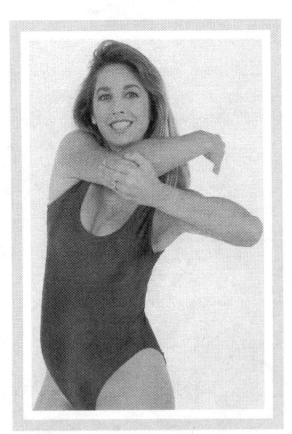

Positive Posture Stretch

Sit cross-legged and raise your arms straight over your head. This stretch elongates the body, giving you a full body reach.

Inhale. Hold for 5 seconds and release, exhaling.

REPEAT 2 times.

BENEFITS: Increases circulation, improves posture.

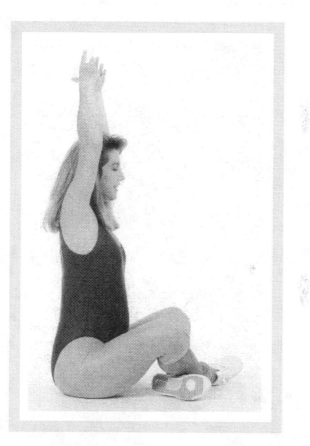

Hips, Thighs, and Buns Stretch

■

Sit on the floor. Bend your knees and pick up one leg. Feel the stretch in the back of the thigh and buttocks. Hold for 10 seconds and release. Switch legs and repeat. You can also roll slowly from side to side to feel all your muscles working.

REPEAT 2 times on each leg.

BENEFITS: Excellent tension reliever. This exercise stretches the pariformus, a muscle that sometimes causes sciatic pain when tight.

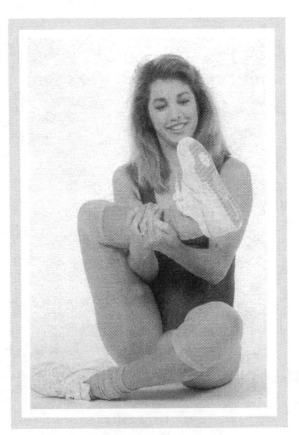

Lower Back Stretch

Get on your knees and, crouching slightly, extend your arms straight out in front of you. Slowly rock back to sit on heels. As your baby grows, move your knees wider apart. While sitting back, walk fingers forward, stretching your arms. Hold for 20 seconds.

BENEFITS: Upper body stretch and lower back extensions. Some people even say this position can turn a breach baby around.

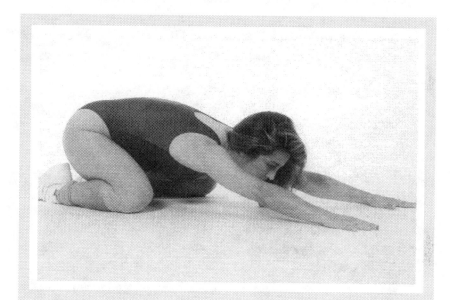

Beauty Tip

If you've never worn foundation or concealer, consider it now. Thanks to an increased blood flow that dilates tiny capillaries during pregnancy, you may experience more blemishes and blotchiness due to hormonal surges. (So much for the glow of pregnancy!) Wear a nice light foundation or tinted moisturizer to even out your skin tone. Keep colors natural and clear. After all, you're a mom-to-be. Save the trendy look for later. This doesn't mean you have to look dowdy. Makeup and motherhood can happily coexist! Like exercise and a good eating plan, makeup is an upper. It makes us feel pretty, and we need to begin to take more time out to feel pretty and good about ourselves.

Beauty Tip

I remember discovering a small brown discoloration on my face around my nose and upper lip area, and it looked as though I had a mustache. The second time around I wore a good sunscreen whenever I was exposed to the sun's rays. During pregnancy sun exposure can send hormone-infused pigment cells into overdrive, triggering dark patches on your face (called the "mask of pregnancy"), so be sure to wear a good sunscreen during the day.

Part Two

Second Trimester

CHAPTER FOUR

Welcome to the Second Trimester

Congratulations! You are now officially four months pregnant, and you are over the hump. Eighty percent of pregnancy losses occur in the first trimester, so you should now be feeling more secure and less anxious. Do you feel like a new person? As if a cloud has lifted? By now your nausea has probably subsided. At least I hope so. (But don't feel bad if it hasn't; some of my friends suffered from morning sickness throughout their entire pregnancies. Hopefully you won't!)

You are now entering the most glorious time of your pregnancy. This period was when I really began to feel like myself again. You should have a little more energy. Those afternoon naps won't be as necessary as before. The change was almost immediate for me, and it signaled the beginning of the easiest time of my pregnancy. My appetite had definitely returned, and I actually savored food again.

It was also an exciting time for Jeff. Now that I was "showing" a little bit, we began to discuss names for the baby. Jeff would laugh at me if we went to a party and I saw women with cute little waistlines. I couldn't wait to be able to wear a belt again. During my first pregnancy I was concerned; would I ever get my rock-hard tummy back?

Jeff kept saying I looked great—even though I had gained seven pounds and totally lost my waistline—and that I would bounce back. I

> *Nothing is a sacrifice if it is done out of love for another person.*

also finally had the energy and desire to have sex again. My doctor assured me that making love was safe. This was a very romantic time for both of us, as we dreamed together of the family we both always wanted.

But something was bothering me at the beginning of my second trimester. I had to tell the bosses at ESPN that I was pregnant.

I kept thinking, Why would they want me now? They'll find someone else. I thought my whole career would be over, everything I had worked so hard for. It had been my dream, and now I thought it might end.

I was scheduled to sit down with the bigwigs at ESPN (all men) to discuss their new lineup of television shows, and I was convinced they wouldn't want to renew my contract. I tossed and turned in bed at night for at least a week before my meeting, my stomach churning.

I had to convince them that *Getting Fit with Denise Austin* should remain on ESPN. Of course, no one at ESPN knew I was pregnant. My only solution was to try to hide the pregnancy, since I didn't want it to be a focal point until after the meeting.

I found the perfect "disguise": a baggy, double-breasted jacket and short skirt. I also invested in a pair of beautiful earrings to draw attention to my face and away from my waistline.

On the day of the meeting, I anxiously dressed and arrived at the studio for my meeting. They were thrilled with my TV show and told me *Getting Fit* was rated number one. They instantly renewed the show for another year. I then felt I had to let them know, and I blurted out that I was five months pregnant!

The ESPN executives were amazed, and delighted. Here I had spent weeks worrying about my future, and they assured me that they not only had faith in my professional work, but they knew that pregnancy or not, every show would be delivered on time (which they were!).

Do we create our own stress? Do we all suffer at one time or another from a case of the what ifs? Of course. In my mind I was sure the ESPN executives would not want a pregnant host of a fitness show. In their minds I was still Denise Austin, and nothing about me had changed (just my shape, ha, ha!).

It just goes to show that you will always be more aware of your body than anyone else, and also, *at the right time,* don't be afraid to tell your

There is medical evidence that stress and anxiety cause the hormonal glands to release adrenaline, which raises your blood pressure and heart rate. Chronic stress can lead to hypertension and heart problems. The opposite is also true. Positive, loving feelings can be good for the heart. The bottom line? Your body does not run efficiently when under stress. So wear a smile and think happy thoughts!

boss you're pregnant. I could never even have imagined how supportive these ESPN executives would be and how simple it was to finally admit my condition!

Of course, it did help that by this time I really started to feel great. My energy level was back. That old "morning sickness" was gone. I got back into my normal exercise routine, which meant a brisk, thirty-to-forty-five-minute walk at least three days a week.

Make every day count. Life is not a dress rehearsal. It's the real thing.

I walked as fast as I could, while pumping my arms. Two days a week I continued my toning routine, doing exercises for twenty to thirty minutes. I did my light weight routine, biceps and tricep exercises, leg lifts, lunges and squats for hips, and thighs and buns and finished with easy stretches.

I remember being invited to a state dinner at the White House during this time, and I was so worried about finding a dress to wear. This is a difficult stage to find good clothes. You're not quite ready for real maternity clothes, but you've grown out of your regular ones. When I went shopping, I couldn't find a maternity evening dress that fit, so I decided to buy a regular dress two sizes larger than my usual size.

It was a great, low-cut, beaded black dress (size ten!). President Bush introduced me to the prime minister of Italy, saying, "This is our good friend Denise. She jumps up and down on television and keeps America fit." You can imagine the Italian translation of that! I met Frank Sinatra, Lee Iacocca, and Elizabeth Taylor, along with all the top White House officials, and I was thrilled to be there, even if I couldn't

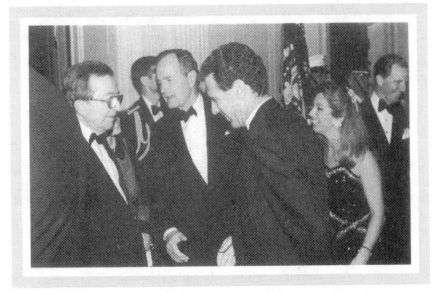

Enjoying ourselves at a State Dinner at the White House while I was five months pregnant with Kelly.

drink the champagne. Everyone said they were shocked to learn I was five months pregnant. The most fun part was that for the first time in my life I actually felt I had cleavage, since I'm normally flat as a board. (I believe in the Wonderbra now!)

I invested in two one-piece maternity bathing suits. Two-piece suits are okay for some mothers-to-be, but I never wore them. My belly button stuck out too much.

I could still wear my same blue jeans, but since I couldn't zip them up all the way, I would take a rubber band and put it through the loop and the top button to fasten the pants.

I also wore bike shorts and cut the elastic in places all around the band to make them fit. Same with my leggings, even my tights and nylons.

Could people tell I was pregnant while I was wearing a leotard, with a loose T-shirt wrapped around my side? I filmed my TV show without saying I was pregnant because the show would run again even after I had the baby. I have to confess it did hurt my feelings when I received some letters asking if I had gained a lot of weight! I thought, If they only knew I was pregnant. I receive four hundred letters each week, and only a few asked, but a lot of women guessed anyhow since my tummy was noticeable, even though I didn't think it was that big. But TV does add ten pounds to how you look.

For business meetings I wore longer double-breasted jackets with the same color skirt. Tip: Wearing all one color makes you look longer and leaner.

I paid special attention to my legs during pregnancy. I adore short skirts.

Give yourself some credit. By now you have been carrying your baby for half its term. A new life is inside you!

LEGS

Your poor aching feet! Your shoes probably feel too tight. (Try buying new shoes one-half size larger during pregnancy.) Now is the time to take a few minutes, after work or before bedtime, to soak them in warm, sudsy water, sprinkle some talcum powder on them, and elevate them often. This is also the perfect time to ask your husband for a foot rub!

For a good foot refresher, all you need is a minute and a tennis ball.

1. Take off your shoes and socks.
2. Place a tennis ball under one foot.
3. Roll the ball back and forth under the foot for 30 seconds.
4. Switch feet and repeat.

KEEPING YOUR BACK HEALTHY DURING PREGNANCY

Nothing can be more debilitating than being pregnant and having your back go out. Now you're bedridden and in pain, and you really can't take any pain relievers. Back injuries are easier to prevent than treat. Here are some back-saving tips for the second trimester:

1. When traveling, divide your stuff into two smaller suitcases instead of one large one. (Don't exert yourself carrying heavy loads.) Two smaller cases will also give you better balance. (This is good advice even if you're not pregnant.)

2. Now's the time to clean out your purse. Some women's purses weigh up to four pounds! That puts tremendous strain on the back and shoulders. When going to the store or running errands, take only the essentials.

3. If you carry a shoulder bag, alternate the weight by carrying the purse on the opposite side every other day. This is all to keep your back muscles in balance. Buy a backpack instead of a purse. Backpacks are in style, cute, and functional.

4. When you are carrying something heavy or lifting a baby, bend your knees. Don't turn or twist abruptly when holding something in your arms. When you are lifting, tighten your abs (even though you can't suck them in). There is nothing worse than lower back pain when you're pregnant.

5. Good posture is of the utmost importance now that you're pregnant. Sit up tall and straight and stand erect with perfect posture.

6. Now is the time to trade in the highest heels for lower ones. I prefer a two-inch heel. But pregnant or not, my first choice is always sneakers.

Dear Denise

I have just discovered several varicose veins on the backs of thighs and calves. Is this normal during pregnancy?

Yes. Chances are if your mother had them, you will, too. Research shows that varicose veins—as well as other complications like high blood pressure—are hereditary during pregnancy. I used to wear support hose during airplane trips to hold everything in.

Circulation exercises are important. Elevate your feet, and the support hose does help. During pregnancy sitting at your desk for prolonged periods of time can lead to back pain and varicose veins and increase the likelihood of blood clots as blood pools in the legs. Standing for long periods can also be hard on you; it decreases blood flow to the uterus.

Water exercise is terrific if you have varicose veins or a sore lower back. It's a *great* workout, burns calories, and is lots of fun.

If you must sit for several hours, get up and stretch at least a few minutes each hour. Go to the bathroom often. Instead of crossing your legs, sit with your feet up on a footrest or open drawer to reduce swelling and take the strain off your back.

Remember, if one knee is higher than your hip level, it helps eliminate back pain.

Stand up and stretch every hour, reaching your arms over your head, to improve circulation and help prevent back pain.

Want to prevent cramps in your calves? Don't point your toes in bed. Remember to flex your foot, toe toward knee, for a good stretch that will elongate the calf muscle. Don't point your toes rigidly; this might cramp and contract your calf muscles. If you do get leg cramps, do not rub your legs. This may increase the cramp. Instead, hold a calf stretch (or grab your toes and pull them back toward your knee).

Don't neglect your safety and your baby's safety in the car. Remember to wear your seat belt at all times. The shoulder strap can go between your breasts, and the lap belt should go underneath your abdomen.

SKIN

By the second trimester you will probably find that your skin is not as temperamental. But something else may happen. Patches of darker skin may begin to appear across your nose and cheeks. I got dark patches on my upper lip, especially after exposure to the sun. Known as *chloasma,* this skin change (which used to be called "the mask of pregnancy") is nothing to worry about. I always used a good skin block and a concealer if I thought I needed it.

AMNIOCENTESIS

During my first pregnancy I did not have amnio. When I became pregnant for the second time, I was over thirty-five, and my doctor recommended I take this test, which is used to determine certain birth defects. The doctor inserts a thin needle into the uterus and takes a sample of your amniotic fluid.

I had the amnio in my sixteenth week with my second child. Jeff came with me. We were excited to see the baby's movements on the sonogram. It is not a painful process, but I did feel a slight sense of discomfort. Afterward my doctor wanted me to take it easy for twenty-four hours, so I stayed home from work that afternoon and avoided exercising for several days. I did feel a little cramping that evening, but it was nothing to be concerned about; by the next day it went away. I had to take a flight to California to be on *The Leeza Show*. I appeared on the program and showed pregnancy exercises.

Two weeks later the doctor called with the results: Everything was fine. It was a huge relief. During my first pregnancy, since I did not have an amnio, I didn't know the sex of my baby (my doctor knew by ultrasound, but I had forbidden him from telling me); I wanted to be surprised. It was so hard, because I kept wanting to peek at my chart during my doctor's appointments.

The second time around, my husband and I were both dying to know the sex of our child. Since I wasn't as nauseated during the first trimester, I thought for sure I was having a boy; it was so different. But they said, "You're having a little girl." We didn't tell anyone, just kept it our secret. Ironically, everyone who saw me swore I was having a boy. It looked like a little basketball sticking out from my tummy. But I have to admit now, looking back, that to be surprised at the moment of birth is much more exciting. In my experience, it was so much more fun to wait for that magic moment in the delivery room when they announce, "It's a . . ."

But having three sisters myself, I was truly grateful that Kelly could have a little sister. My sisters mean the world to me. But of course, whatever you have is God's will, and the health of your baby is much more important than anything else.

DON'T FEEL EMBARRASSED if you are absentminded. This is a normal part of pregnancy. I forgot things, too. But just wait until motherhood, when your child expects you to remember *everything*—where they put their shoes, backpack, favorite toy, and so on.

Research shows that your baby begins to recognize human voices by the fifth month. Brush up now on the words to "Ba Ba Black Sheep" and other soothing nursery rhymes. It's also a great way for you to relax.

These are the best months of your pregnancy. Enjoy it while you can! Take advantage of every moment. Take your vacation now (while you still can fly) or indulge in a romantic weekend.

SECOND TRIMESTER HEALTH QUESTIONS

Q. *Is it safe to take long, hot baths and saunas now?*

A. *No. Your body cannot handle the high temperatures of long, steaming hot baths, saunas, and particularly hot tubs. Pregnant women should avoid* overheating their bodies for extended periods. Throughout your pregnancy saunas can be dangerous to you and your baby.

Q. *Is there any way to prevent stretch marks?*

A. *Not really. Chances are if your mother had stretch marks while carrying you, you will probably get them, too. This is normal. Stretch marks are caused by the stretching of the skin due to the large and/or rapid increase in weight. The best preventive is not to gain too much weight during your pregnancy. That's another reason I encourage exercise and nutrition. Expectant mothers with good elastic tone (through years of exercise) may not notice any stretch marks. I was one of the lucky ones, thanks to years of being fit and staying in shape. But several of my friends did get stretch marks. The good news is they fade to a silvery sheen after birth. Another badge of motherhood!*

While I was pregnant, I used lots of moisturizers and lotions on my body, especially immediately after the shower. The cream helped lock in moisture on my body. I also took vitamin E capsules, poked them open, and rubbed them on my expanding tummy. I do think it helped prevent stretch marks. There is no scientific proof, but it worked for me.

DENISE'S TOP TEN PREGNANCY MUSTS

1. Eat a balanced, healthy diet. Strive for five each day: two veggies and three fruits, or three veggies and two fruits.
2. Exercise for health and circulation. Keep on moving! And always check with your doctor before any new routine or activity.
3. Get eight hours of sleep every night.
4. Don't smoke. Avoid alcohol and caffeine and be drug-free.
5. Get early prenatal care. See your doctor for regular checkups.
6. Wear your seat belt.
7. Take five to ten minutes each day for relaxation time. Close your eyes, take a nap, or just calm the body in some way.
8. Drink eight glasses of water each day.
9. Stay in contact with friends and family. . . . Rejoice in the feelings of close connections as you prepare to bring a new life into your world.
10. Keep a positive attitude! Do things that make you happy.

CHAPTER 5

Eating Smart and Happy Snacking

*F*ood, glorious food! At this stage in both of my pregnancies, all I could think of was food. Hot, cold, it didn't even matter if it was on someone else's plate! I wasn't craving noodles and bread anymore. I could eat spicier foods and even started to crave Mexican food. But mostly what I wanted was old-fashioned meals, just like my mom used to make: comfort foods like turkey with all the fixin's; meat loaf and mashed potatoes; green vegetables and scalloped potatoes. If I was going to have a hamburger for dinner, I wanted potatoes and a salad with it. I felt hungry all the time.

This is normal! At this stage in our pregnancies, we have a healthy appetite. It's not unusual to get attached to certain foods. I ate Cream of Wheat every morning for almost a month. I became addicted to tuna fish sandwiches and ate one every day for three weeks straight.

I also craved yogurt, and it became my snack of choice. I made lots of fruit smoothies with yogurt and any fresh fruits I had on hand: strawberries, bananas, sliced peaches.

*S*ome things, like our bone structure, we cannot control. But we do have control over everything we put into our bodies. Choose the best foods to fuel you during your pregnancy and keep your baby running.

For a high-calcium snack, try any of these three delicious drinks:

Strawberry yogurt smoothie: Blend ¼ cup low-fat strawberry yogurt with ½ cup skim milk and ¼ cup fresh or frozen strawberries. Mix in a blender or use a hand mixer. Only 107 calories.

Orange dream delight: Blend ¾ cup orange juice, ½ cup milk, and ¼ teaspoon vanilla. Whir in blender. If not sweet enough, add sugar to taste. Only 110 calories.

Marvelous melon smoothie: Blend 1 cup cubed ripe cantaloupe, ½ cup fat-free vanilla frozen yogurt, 1 tablespoon frozen orange juice concentrate, and 1 ice cube. Mix in blender until smooth. Only 140 calories.

I ALSO LOVED making hearty soups. I used to make a big pot of vegetable soup, and it would last all week long. Peanut-butter sandwiches tasted so good, and I also loved graham crackers with jam or jelly as an evening snack.

Here are some ideas for quick and delicious pick-me-ups.

DENISE'S HAPPY SNACKS

Snacking keeps your energy high, your metabolism revved up, and hunger in check. These are some of my favorites:

- **2 low-fat vanilla wafer sandwiches (4 cookies), each with ½ teaspoon low-fat cream cheese and 1 slice banana**
- **2 tablespoons canned fat-free refried beans, microwaved on one 6-inch corn tortilla**
- **4 slices Melba toast, each spread with 1 teaspoon nonfat cottage cheese with pineapple**
- **2 celery stalks stuffed with low-fat cream cheese and chives**
- **4 cinnamon graham cracker squares, each spread with ½ teaspoon jam**
- **1 box Cracker Jack and ½ glass skim milk with 1 teaspoon chocolate Ovaltine**
- **1 cup baby carrots dipped in nonfat cottage cheese mixed with salsa**

WEIGHT GAIN. HOW MUCH IS TOO MUCH?

I worked my whole life to stay in shape, to be fit and trim. After all, it's my career. So when the pounds started coming (and come they do), I wanted to know what all this extra weight came from food not counting! Now, in the second trimester, is the time for you to be putting on pounds gradually.

By now you too are probably wondering where the pregnancy pounds actually go.

The following chart will help you understand your weight gain.

Maternal stores of fat, protein, and other nutrients	7 pounds
Increased body fluid	4 pounds
Increased blood	3–4 pounds
Breast growth	1–2 pounds
Enlarged uterus	2 pounds
Amniotic fluid	2 pounds
Placenta	1 ½ pounds
Baby	6–8 pounds
Total	26½–30½ pounds

Depending on your prepregnancy weight, your average weight gain from the fourth month on is about one pound per week.

Dear Denise

I am six months pregnant, and I know my stomach is growing, but why is my butt so big?

Don't worry, honey, it's nature's way. You need to keep up good eating habits. Walking will help, and so will certain exercises, but most important, there are medical reasons why your fat is being stored in your hips. Your body is preparing itself for childbirth. Your body needs the extra weight, and your hips are the most efficient place to store the extra fat. But there is good news! That fat is usually the first to go after childbirth, so don't despair.

Dear Denise

I have been trying to lose weight for over a year now, and I just found out I'm pregnant! Is this a cruel trick? I'm thrilled to be having a baby, but I'm worried about the weight gain.

If you are starting out your pregnancy on the heavier side, focus on a well-balanced diet during the first trimester. Now is not the time even to think about losing weight. By the second trimester aim for a gradual weight gain shown in this chart from the National Academy of Sciences. Discuss weight maintenance with your doctor as an option to a weight gain. Your body can lose fat gradually one pound a week, while the baby is gaining one pound a week. Some overweight women have even weighed less after delivery than they did before pregnancy. This can be done safely if you work with your doctor and a licensed nutritionist.

Continue exercising three to five times a week to control your weight, as in any time of your life. Remember, this is only nine months of your life. Give your baby the head start he or she deserves. You *will* get back into shape, I promise!

There are certain guidelines for women to follow, depending on their prepregnancy weight. Underweight women who do not gain enough during pregnancy are in danger of delivering premature or small infants. Women who are of normal weight at the time of pregnancy and go on to gain too much may be candidates for gestational diabetes, high blood pressure, and even preeclampsia (a dangerous condition marked by high blood pressure, fluid retention, and loss of protein through urine).

Underweight women should aim for a gain of twenty-eight to forty pounds.

Normal women should aim for a gain of twenty-five to thirty-five pounds.

Overweight women should aim for a gain of fifteen to twenty-five pounds.

Obese women should aim for a gain of fifteen pounds or less.

PROTEIN

As a fitness expert I get lots of questions about sports nutrition, including ones concerning the benefits of sports drinks and high-protein bars now on the market. Studies have shown that sports drinks containing glucose and sodium may enhance short-term exercise performance. But remember, these drinks are often high in calories. Ideally I would recommend sticking to water.

Athletes generally need more protein than sedentary people, and pregnant exercising women fall into that category. Among sports nutritionists, power bars (also known as "energy bars") have become popular. These quick pick-me-uppers are rich in vitamins and minerals but also high in calories (many of them weigh in at 250 calories—the same as a candy bar!). They are not a substitute for whole foods and cannot really benefit a woman who has a poor diet. Read the labels carefully, and beware false claims. Bars, although a convenient energy source, do not replace a well-balanced meal!

Here is a quick chart to help you identify foods high in protein:

Which Foods?	Grams of Protein?
3½ ounces broiled chicken breast	31 grams
3½ ounces broiled hamburger (or other lean meat)	25 grams
3½-ounce can tuna	24 grams
½ cup cottage cheese	14 grams
1-inch cube cheese	7 grams
1 egg white	6 grams
1 tablespoon peanut butter	4 grams
4 ounces broiled fish	24 grams
4 ounces cottage cheese (low-fat)	17 grams
1 cup skim milk	8 grams
4 ounces beans	15 grams
1 potato	5 grams
3 ounces turkey	20 grams

By fifteen weeks I had gained 10 pounds and weighed 127 pounds. Looking at my doctor's chart, I saw that I gained the exact same amount with both pregnancies, and at about the same time.

I also began craving certain foods and knew that I would quickly gain more weight if I couldn't control these cravings. Remember, it's okay to give in once in a while to temptation. But it also helps to have alternatives on hand in your pantry or kitchen.

Here are a few of my crave stoppers that will help you curb your cravings, too.

If you want something chocolate, try . . .

¾ cup Dannon Light chocolate frozen yogurt

½ cup 1 percent chocolate milk

2 chocolate rice cakes

Note: Remember, chocolate contains caffeine, so beware!

If you want something salty and crunchy try . . .

1 ounce pretzels

9 saltine crackers

4 cups low-fat microwave popcorn

5 no-fat-added whole-wheat crackers

If you want something sweet, try . . .

Life Savers or Good & Plenty licorice candy: no fat!

Frozen fruit juice bar

Small slice of angel food cake

8 animal crackers

If you want something creamy, try . . .

¾ cup applesauce

½ cup skim milk pudding

1 cup low-fat or no-fat yogurt

½ cup fat-free ice cream

½ cup low-fat cottage cheese

During both of my pregnancies, I experienced a little constipation from time to time, but it was normal and expected. Because of the hormones in your body, elimination becomes a little less efficient. Pressure from the uterus on the bowels can also cause irregularity.

Make sure to add more fiber to your diet. Eat more vegetables and fruit. I recommend raisins, prunes, apricots, whole-grain cereals, and breads.

Denise's daily dose: For a great natural stool softener that you can drink every day, mix equal amounts of prune juice, apricot juice, and orange juice. Drink half a cup each day.

And remember to drink your water! Eight glasses each day.

Diet tip . . . Certain foods are high in water content and can contribute to your daily intake. They are oranges, melons, tomatoes, and strawberries. Avoid bananas, as they are quite constipating.

Meal Plan for Constipation

Second trimester: As the baby starts to grow, you may feel more uncomfortable owing partially to expanded growth of your midsection as well as to hormonal changes that relax muscles to accommodate your expanding uterus. These changes can also cause intestinal movements to slow down, causing constipation. Here is a meal plan to help:

Breakfast

¾ cup oatmeal with 2 tablespoons raisins

½ grapefruit

8 ounces skim milk

8 ounces water

Midmorning

1 pear

8 ounces seltzer water

Lunch

Gardenburger with 1 slice mozzarella cheese melted on
top, lettuce, and tomato on a whole-grain bun

1 apple

2 fig bars

8 ounces water

Midafternoon

6-ounce container fruit-flavored low-fat yogurt

8 ounces seltzer or lemon water

Dinner

4 ounces pork tenderloin (raw weight 5 ounces) sautéed
in a pan sprayed with vegetable spray and sautéed
with onions, apple juice, and rosemary (about
20 minutes, or until no longer pink)

1 baked potato (with skin) and 1 tablespoon
whipped butter

½ cup steamed peas

8 ounce glass lemon water

Total

Calories: 1,952

Fat: 47 grams

Fiber: 30 grams

Carbohydrate 58 percent, Protein 22 percent,
Fat 20 percent

Q. *I've just been diagnosed with a mild case of anemia. Does this mean I have to stop exercising?*

A. *No. Most doctors will recommend more rest for a pregnant woman with a mild case of anemia, but there's no reason to restrict your activities, as long as you feel up to it and don't get overtired. In most cases anemia is temporary and can be cured with diet and mineral supplements.*

Anemia—which tends to occur around the twentieth week of pregnancy— results from a low level of hemoglobin, which carries oxygen to the body through your red blood cells. It is caused by lack of iron and folic acid in your diet. Even if you're getting enough vitamins and minerals, pregnancy alters the digestive process so the baby can consume some of the iron and folic acid normally available to your body.

Some women don't have any symptoms at all. In more serious cases a woman might experience weakness or fainting, pale skin color, and breathlessness. To prevent anemia, choose foods rich in iron (liver, beef, whole-grain breads), folic acid (beans, wheat germ, broccoli, and asparagus), and vitamin C (citrus fruits and fresh raw veggies). Vitamin C helps your body absorb iron.

Note: If your doctor prescribes an iron supplement, it's best to take it one hour before eating or between meals. Drink plenty of fluids to avoid constipation.

Iron tip . . . Some researchers have found that cooking with the old-fashioned cast-iron skillets and kettles (the black ones, not enamelled) can actually increase your iron absorption. Acid-rich foods like spaghetti sauce can draw the iron into the food, increasing your iron intake by almost 30 percent.

Here are six "comfort foods" I loved during my second trimester.

Denise's Meatloaf

(Serves 4)

∎

1 EGG

½ CUP PEPPERIDGE FARM HERB STUFFING MIX

¾ CUP SKIM MILK

1 TEASPOON OREGANO

1 TABLESPOON CHOPPED PARSLEY

1 SMALL CAN TOMATO SAUCE

1 POUND GROUND TURKEY

½ POUND LEAN GROUND BEEF

Preheat oven to 350 degrees.

Put egg in large bowl and whisk lightly. Add stuffing mix, milk, oregano, parsley, and half can of the tomato sauce. Stir to blend and let sit a minute. Work in ground meat and mix well (I use my hands). Shape into loaf and place into baking dish. Cover with remaining tomato sauce.

Bake for forty minutes.

NOTE: When using dried herbs, never shake them directly into the recipe. Measure out and crush with your fingers to release the flavor before adding.

Yummy Scalloped Potatoes

(Serves 4)

∎

5 RUSSET BAKING POTATOES
1 CUP LIGHT CREAM (OR SUBSTITUTE HALF AND HALF)
1 CUP SKIM MILK
DASH OF NUTMEG
2 TABLESPOONS GRATED GRUYÈRE CHEESE.

Preheat oven to 350 degrees.

Peel potatoes, but do not rinse them (the starch on the potatoes will help thicken the sauce naturally). Slice almost paper thin and pat dry. Put in large pot and cover with the cream and milk. (For a low-fat dish, use all skim milk.) Over low-medium heat, bring potatoes to the boil, stirring once or twice. (Don't let the potatoes burn on the bottom.) Let potatoes boil for two minutes. Take off heat, add nutmeg, stir, and transfer potatoes into a casserole dish, top with sprinkled cheese, and bake for forty minutes, or until top is browned and bubbly.

NOTE: Sometimes I rub the bottom of the dish with a cut clove of garlic to give the potatoes extra flavor.

Rosemary Roasted Chicken with Crispy Potatoes

(Serves 4)

■

2-POUND ROASTING CHICKEN
2 TABLESPOONS OLIVE OIL
3 TABLESPOONS FRESH OR DRIED ROSEMARY
4–5 RUSSET BAKING POTATOES
5 TABLESPOONS OLIVE OIL
1 TABLESPOON BUTTER OR MARGARINE
SALT AND FRESH GROUND PEPPER TO TASTE

Preheat oven to 400 degrees.

Wash chicken inside and out and pat dry. Rub with 2 tablespoons olive oil and one tablespoon of the rosemary. Put the remaining 2 tablespoons rosemary inside the chicken cavity.

Place chicken, breast side up, in shallow dish and roast for ten minutes.

After ten minutes reduce the heat to 350 degrees and turn the chicken over, breast side down. Continue roasting, basting once or twice.

Meanwhile, peel baking potatoes, rinse, and quarter. Pat dry.

In a large casserole or Dutch oven, heat 5 tablespoons olive oil over medium heat. Add potatoes and sauté until nicely browned. Drain off the oil and dot the potatoes with butter or margarine. Season with salt and pepper to taste.

You can either add the potatoes to the chicken roasting pan or bake them in a separate dish for forty minutes or until nicely browned.

The chicken and the crispy potatoes should be done at the same time.

Tuscan Bean Soup

(Serves 4)

■

4 CLOVES GARLIC, MINCED
1/4 CUP OLIVE OIL
2 19-OUNCE CANS CANNELLINI BEANS,
DRAINED OF LIQUID
3 CUPS DEFATTED VEAL OR CHICKEN STOCK
SALT AND PEPPER TO TASTE

In a heavy-bottomed soup pot or Dutch oven, sauté garlic in olive oil over low heat until golden. Add beans, stir, and cover pot. Turn heat to medium and simmer until beans are tender, about ten minutes. Stir once or twice. Turn off heat, transfer beans to food processor, and puree until smooth. Return bean mixture to the pot, add the broth, and simmer for another five minutes. Serve with little garlic toasts or croutons. Sometimes I like to garnish with a few snips of fresh basil, if I have some on hand.

NOTE: I used canned beans for this recipe, since they are more convenient, but if you want to use dried cannellini beans, simply follow the directions on the package, cook, and drain. Proceed with recipe.

"Almost Like Mom's" Macaroni & Cheese

(Serves 5)

BOX OF MACARONI
$\frac{1}{2}$ CUP LIGHT CREAM
$1\frac{1}{2}$ CUPS SKIM MILK
2 TABLESPOONS CORNSTARCH
SALT AND PEPPER
DASH OF WORCESTERSHIRE SAUCE
1 CUP SHREDDED REDUCED-FAT CHEDDAR CHEESE
(SHARP OR EXTRA SHARP)
BREAD CRUMBS OR LOW-FAT CRACKERS CRUMBLED
IN FOOD PROCESSOR (FOR TOPPING)

Cook macaroni according to directions on the package, drain, and set aside. In a large skillet, whisk cream and milk with cornstarch until dissolved. Cook over low to medium heat, stirring often, until thickened. Add seasonings and cheese and transfer mixture to a casserole dish. Top with bread crumbs. Serve right away or refrigerate, covered. To reheat, bake at 350 degrees until top is brown and bubbly, about ten minutes.

Old-Fashioned Fruit Cobbler

(Serves 4)

You can use almost any fruit or combination of fruits for the following recipe. I like peaches, strawberries, and blueberries, but you can use raspberries, pears, apples, canned or frozen cherries, or whatever you have on hand.

2 RIPE PEACHES, PEELED AND SLICED
1 PINT BLUEBERRIES, WASHED AND PICKED OVER
½ PINT STRAWBERRIES, SLICED
JUICE OF 1 LEMON
½ CUP LIGHT BROWN SUGAR
¾ CUP FLOUR
2 TABLESPOONS BUTTER OR MARGARINE

Preheat oven to 350 degrees.

Place fruit in an ovenproof casserole dish. In a separate bowl, mix flour, sugar, and butter together. Spoon batter over fruit and bake for twenty-five minutes, or until top is brown and bubbly.

Serve plain or with low-fat vanilla yogurt or ice cream.

SECOND TRIMESTER NUTRITION QUESTIONS

Q. *Do I really need to be eating for two?*

A. *Eating for two does not mean eating two adult portions at every meal. The goal is to gain a healthy amount of weight, not to put on so many pounds that it will be a struggle to get them off after the baby is born. Think of it as eating healthfully for one, without junk or empty calories. You will gain the weight the baby needs, with all the essential nutrients, but will have an easier time with your after-baby shape-up. Don't set yourself up for frustration. I know appetites are heartier now, but you need to be moderate in portion control.*

Portion control tips: Think of four ounces (usually considered one serving) of meat, poultry, or fish as the size of a deck of cards. Think of ½ cup of fruit as the size of a tennis ball. Two tablespoons of peanut butter are the size of a golf ball. Two ounces of pretzels should fit into the palm of your hand. I always like to remember that one tablespoon is equivalent to the first joint of my thumb.

CHAPTER 6

You Can Do It! Exercises for the Second Trimester

Warm-up

Put on your favorite music and begin to march in place. Raise your legs, and gently pump your arms in time to the beat. It's time to get your blood pumping; get started: march in place or walk for 3 minutes.

BENEFITS: Increases blood circulation, burns a few calories, and gets your ready for the tone-up routine. Plus, it gets the oxygen flowing!

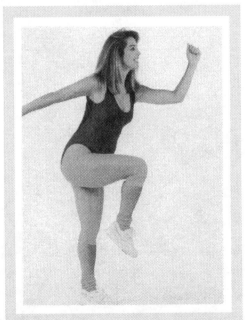

Plié

•

If you feel that your balance is slightly off, use a chair for this exercise.

Stand with your legs apart. Your feet should be a little wider than your hips. Your feet should be slightly turned out. If using a chair, place your hand on the back for balance. Your back should be straight and your abs tight.

Tilt your pelvis forward and keep your hips square to the front. Bend your knees (keeping the knees traveling over your toes and not beyond) and lower your hips toward the floor. As you come back up, straighten your legs, but don't lock your knees. Exhale and squeeze your buttocks.

REPEAT 2 sets of 8–12 reps each. Rest for 15 seconds between sets.

BENEFITS: Thighs (quadriceps). Don't quit! Our legs need to stay in shape to ward off fat deposits.

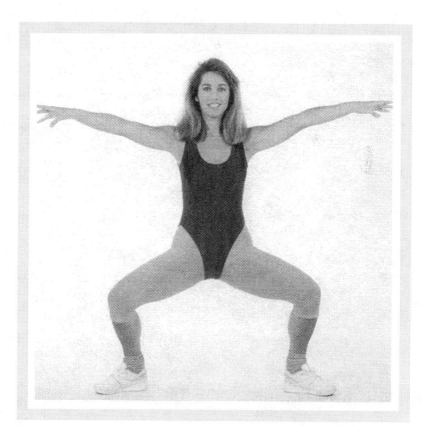

Triceps Toner

■

Fight that underarm sag and flab. We'll firm up with this exercise designed to tone up the upper-back part of your arms and your triceps. Tightening these muscles will help you eliminate that jiggle on the back of your arms. If you have been using light weights, continue to do so. During the second trimester you can even make strength gain. Go for it, but don't overdo it!

Stand up with your left leg in front of your right and bend the left knee slightly. Keep your arm bent. Keep your abs tight and your back flat. Raise your right elbow so that the upper part of your arm is parallel with the floor. Keep your elbow close to your body. Straighten your right arm. Be sure to squeeze your triceps as you straighten your arm.

Return your right hand to the starting position, pause, and repeat the movement.

VARIATION: Straighten your right arm as shown. Hold a weight in your hand, and don't be afraid to lighten your load or put it down if it feels too heavy.

REPEAT 2 sets, 8–12 times.

BENEFITS: Firms the triceps and strengthens the arms for future baby lifting and holding. We want to avoid using our back to pick up the baby.

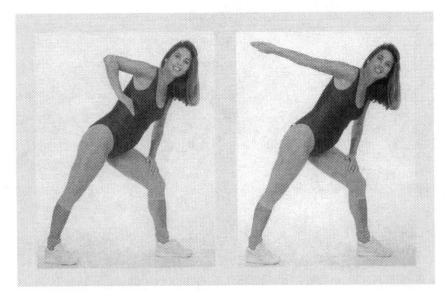

Baby Lunge

·

The best exercise for your bottom half! Start with your feet about shoulder-width apart. Take a step backward with one foot. Make sure your front knee stays at a ninety-degree angle. Keep your knee in line with your ankle. Your ligaments are looser and more prone to injury now, so make sure you don't lock your knee. As you step back, bend your back knee. Be sure you don't touch your back knee on the floor. Your weight should be balanced between your back toes and your front heel.

Push back to the starting position, bringing legs together, and repeat, alternating your legs.

REPEAT 2 sets of 8–12 reps each. Rest 15 seconds between sets.

BENEFITS: Thighs (quadriceps), hamstrings, buttocks.

Keeps your entire lower body toned.

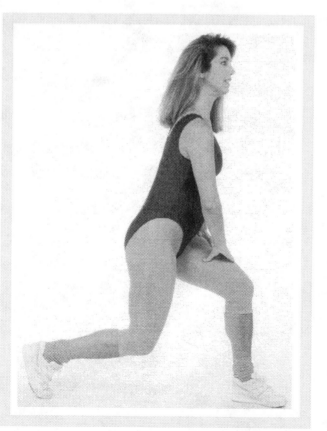

Chest Firmer

We must pay attention to our growing bust! Keep them firm and "lifted."

Extend your arms to the side, elbows bent so that your fingers point inward. Bring your forearms together in front of your chest, maintaining resistance. Press your arms back out again, keeping the muscles tight. Do a modified arm scissors movement, with your arms slightly bent.

REPEAT 2 sets of 8–12 reps.

BENEFITS: Strengthens upper chest muscles.

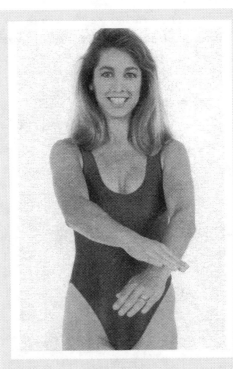

Thigh Shaper

■

Sit on the floor and place one hand on your knee. Lift your leg, being careful not to point your toes too rigidly. Keep your leg straight, but don't lock your knees. Lift and lower your leg 5 inches up, then slowly lower back down.

REPEAT 2 sets of 8–12 leg lifts on each leg.

BENEFITS: Tones thighs, abs, and hip flexor. This exercise keeps the muscles surrounding your knees strong to protect your knee joints. Also great to firm up flabby knees.

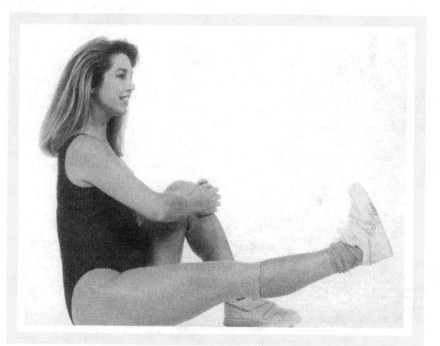

Hip Slimmer

Great one for your hips and outer thighs. Lie on your side. You might want to place a pillow under your head for comfort. Bend your knee underneath your body. Keep the other leg straight on top, with your arm outstretched.

Keeping your leg straight and your foot flexed, raise your leg slowly. Lower it back to the floor, then repeat. Be careful not to raise your leg too high. Keep your knee facing forward. You should be focusing on the outer thigh of your top leg.

REPEAT 2 sets of 8–12 legs lifts on each leg.

BENEFITS: Outer thigh (abductors). Helps keep pregnant hips from "spreading."

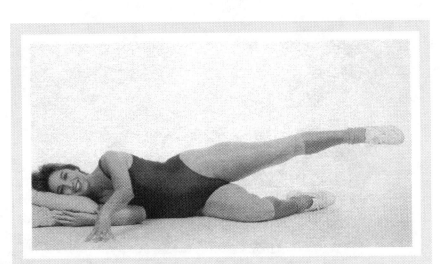

Hip Rock

Great for abdominal strength and lower back stretching. On your hands and knees, swivel your hips from left to right, tightening your abdominal muscles. Don't let your tummy sag. Lift and pull in your abs as you rock slightly.

REPEAT 2 sets of 8–12 reps. Rest for 15 seconds between sets.

BENEFITS: Excellent for abdominal strengthening. Increases flexibility in your trunk and hips.

Note: Four weeks before giving birth to Kelly I was advised to do this exercise after it was determined that my baby was in the breech position. The doctor confirmed that she had completely turned, so it worked!

During labor my nurse asked me to do this exercise to help relieve back pain, and it did help a little.

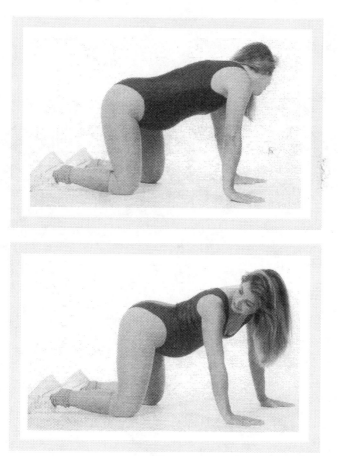

Upper-Body Strengthener

One of the best exercises you could ever do to strengthen your upper body is a push-up. Place your body weight on your knees and hands. You are going to do a modified push-up by slowly lowering your hands and chest to the floor, bending your elbows. Push up by straightening your elbows and then return to the starting position. Keep your abs tight.

One easier variation of this exercise is to stand against a wall and lean your body forward and push back.

REPEAT 2 sets of 8–12 reps each. Rest 15 seconds between sets.

BENEFITS: Chest (pectorals), shoulders (anterior deltoid), triceps.

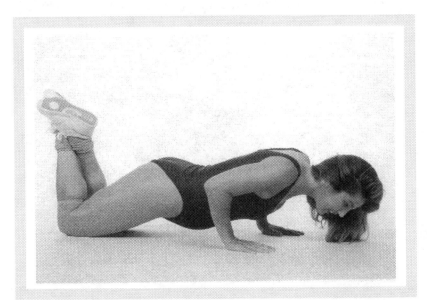

Thigh and Tush Tightener

.

Have a great rear view while pregnant—seeing you from behind, they won't even know you're pregnant! Kneel on the floor with both elbows directly under your shoulders, your left knee under your left hip, and hands on the floor. Straighten the right leg behind you, with toes resting on the floor. Keep your back flat, your abs tight, and your hips square to the floor. Keeping your right leg straight, use your buttocks to lift the entire leg up. Now, lower the leg. Slowly raise your leg up and down for 2 sets. Do not arch your back, and *squeeze* the buttocks. If you feel dizzy, nauseous, or light-headed, perform this exercise on your hands, not your elbows.

REPEAT 2 sets of 8–12 reps per leg. Rest 15 seconds between sets.

BENEFITS: Make your bottom half your better half! Since your tummy is getting bigger, make sure your legs look their best.

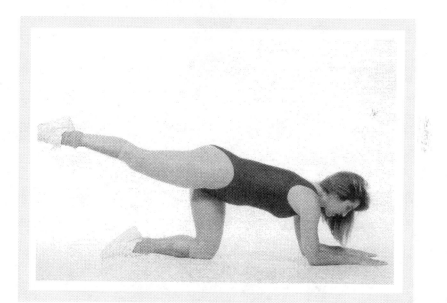

Calf Stretch

.

This is a great muscle cramp reliever.

Place one foot in front of the other. Bend your front knee and support your hands on your thigh. Keep your back heel flat on the floor, holding the stretch for 10–15 seconds.

REPEAT 2 sets of 8–12 reps.

BENEFITS: Stretches lower legs and relieves achy muscles.

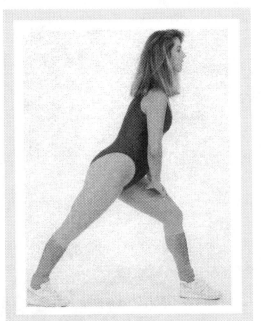

*L*ook for ways to get extra rest. Go to bed early, or take naps during the day. You're working hard to build a new human, and that takes energy.

Modified Situp for Moms-to-Be

.

Q. *Why are pregnant women told not to exercise on their backs after twelve weeks (your first trimester)?*

A. *Exercising on your back may put pressure on your inferior vena cava, the vein that returns blood from the legs and torso to the heart. Pressure on this vein can result in hypotension (abnormally low blood pressure), which can cause dizziness, nausea, and shortness of breath. This doesn't have to eliminate abdominal strengthening. There are ways to modify a situp and still strengthen your abs safely during pregnancy.*

I did modify my abdominal exercises by the fourth month of pregnancy. Pregnant women should not do any exercises on their back. But of course I wanted to keep my abdominals strong, so here are some great second trimester abdominal exercises to do to keep your abs strong and your back healthy. Since your abs and back will be "holding your baby," they are the "core" of your whole body and need to stay strong.

Maternity Situps: After sixteen weeks, we are no longer allowed to do any exercises on our backs. The following four exercises—my "patented" special personal tummy exercises—are alternatives to the traditional situp and will help strengthen your abdominal muscles . . . which is so important.

Standing Tummy Tuck

■

Stand with your feet shoulder-width apart. Bend your knees and put your hands on your thighs to support your back. Your back should be flat. Take a deep breath and round your back and pull in and tighten your abdominals, exhaling out. Then release to a natural flat back position.

REPEAT 5 times, holding the stretch for 3–4 seconds.

BENEFITS: Strengthens abdominals, stretches lower back.

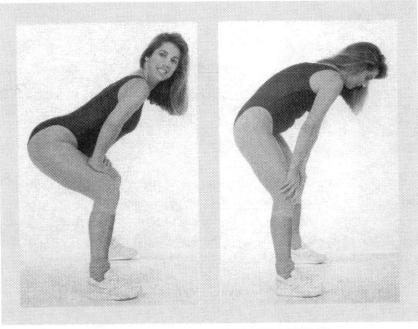

INHALE.   EXHALE AND TIGHTEN ABS.

Standing Pelvic Tilt

.

Stand with your knees slightly bent. Stand nice and tall. Think "good posture"! Curl your buttocks in and tilt your pelvis forward. Tighten up your abs and your tush, holding them for five seconds, and release.

REPEAT 10 times.

BENEFITS: Improves posture, strengthens abdominals, and relieves pressure from your back muscles.

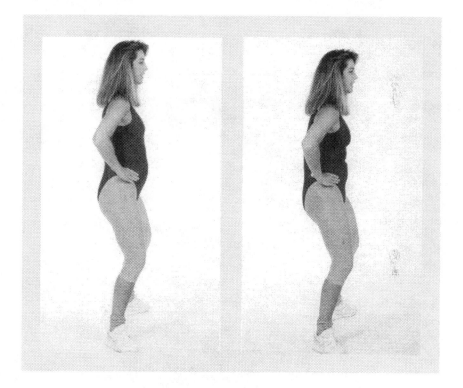

"Expectant" Ab Exercise

Kneel on all fours, being careful not to let your stomach sag. Inhale deeply and as you slowly roll up your back into an arch position, exhale and tighten your abdominal muscles. Hold for 3–4 seconds. Release and repeat. Don't put too much pressure on your wrists. Alternate using your knuckles or fingertips.

REPEAT 2 sets of 8–12 reps.

BENEFITS: Strengthens abdominals.

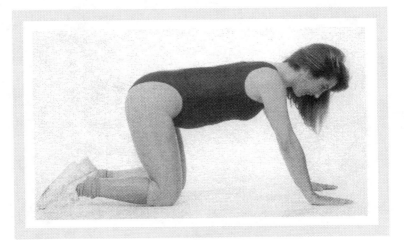

INHALE.

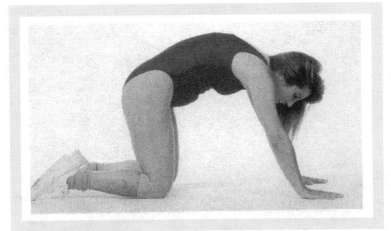

EXHALE AND TIGHTEN ABS.

Seated Tummy Tightener

Sit on the floor with your knees bent and back straight. Place your hands underneath your thighs to support your back. Slowly roll back, contracting your abdominals and exhaling. Inhale as you sit back up straight.

REPEAT 2 sets of 8–12 reps.

BENEFITS: Helps to stabilize your back and strengthen abdominal muscles.

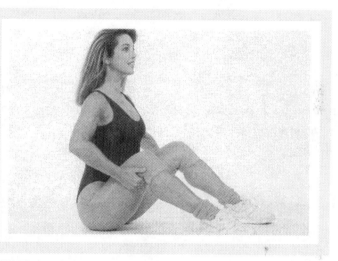

INHALE.

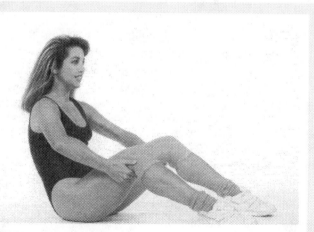

EXHALE AND TIGHTEN ABS.

Q. *I've heard that pregnancy causes loose ligaments and that pregnant women are more prone to injury. Is this true?*

A. *The pregnancy hormone relaxin loosens the ligaments of the pelvis (widening the pelvis up to twelve millimeters in preparation for giving birth). The rib cage also expands about 2–4 inches to accommodate the growing baby. A recent study showed that excessive joint flexibility occurred in pregnant women's knee joints, reaching a peak just before the fifth month of pregnancy.*

Pregnant women should be cautious of injury only because they are placing more body weight on the joints, and balance is off. So be careful!

Q. *What should my target heart rate be during aerobics?*

A. *The old ACOG guidelines required the heart rate to stay under 140 beats per minute. The new ACOG guidelines that were written in 1994 do not have a heart rate restriction. Exercise at a comfortable level for you. If you can talk while you are exercising, you should be fine! I was more cautious and kept my heart rate at 130 beats per minute and kept up my aerobics for thirty to forty minutes, three days a week.*

Remember, aerobics can be anything—walking, biking, swimming—it all counts!

Q. *I've just been told I have separation of the abdominal muscles. Is this serious?*

A. *The stomach muscles can separate down the center of the abdomen, a condition known as diastasis recti. This can be caused by the enlarging baby pushing on the uterine wall, straining a muscle during movements, or hormones. It occurs mainly during the second trimester, and while it is quite normal and not painful, it can be a cause for worry. If the separation is greater than one inch, you will probably want to check with your doctor.*

Q. *Can I continue doing yoga during pregnancy?*

A. *Yoga exercises are perfectly fine to do during pregnancy. In fact, they are a wonderful stress reducer and body firmer. However, one should be careful not to overstretch during pregnancy or postpartum. The hormones in the pregnant woman's body are indiscriminate in their release. This means that those stretching hormones do not just go to the tummy and the chest, they* go everywhere! *You must protect your joints, tendons, and ligaments during pregnancy, so stretch carefully and do not push yourself. If something feels uncomfortable, do not do it.*

In addition, postpartum women should also be careful. The hormones that helped your body to expand and accommodate a growing baby stay in your system for six to eighteen months postpartum! This is how your body will be able to return to its pre-pregnancy shape. These hormones are good. But remember, don't just jump (and I do mean jump*) back into exercise. You still have all these stretching hormones in your system. Walking, toning, water exercise, biking, stair-steppers, step aerobics are all fine to do postpartum. Be careful if you go back to jogging or advanced yoga. Give your body time to return to its pre-pregnancy state, before you risk impact or overstretching injuries.*

Q. *Sometimes during exercise I get a cramp in my side. Is this harmful to the baby?*

A. *No. During exercise, it's not unusual to get a "side stitch," which can be uncomfortable. Over the course of my pregnancies I would sometimes get a cramp in my side if I walked too fast. When I slowed down and took a few breaths, it helped. Also, I would simply massage my side. Make sure to drink enough water before, during, and after exercise. Cramps can also be due to the stretching of the ligaments that support the uterus, and this is nothing to worry about. If cramping is severe, or accompanied by bleeding, be sure to call your doctor.*

Q. *I've heard that women should not continue running during pregnancy. Is this true?*

A. *No. As long as you ran before you became pregnant, you can continue. But now is definitely not the time to start, if you are not experienced. Walking would be better for you.*

While not many of our mothers or grandmothers were into running, it is a popular sport for many women. Ideally pregnancy should not hinder you from continuing to pursue this cardiovascular workout, as long as you are comfortable. Unless your doctor has advised against it, running is a good exercise for pregnant women, with some modification. Studies show that women runners who average twenty-five miles a week have normal deliveries. We've even had pregnant women run a marathon, complete a triathlon, and do a twenty-five-kilometer cross-country ski race!

To run safely, stretch gently as always to prevent injuries. Concentrate on hamstrings, quadriceps, soleus (lower leg), calf muscles, Achilles' and lower back muscles. Pay attention to your body. It will tell when not to push yourself. As with any exercise, if there is pain, stop. Remember, moderation is the key.

Dear Denise,

I'm continuing to walk in my second trimester. Sometimes I get short of breath. Is this normal?

Yes. It's normal to feel breathless sometimes during or after exercise. The pressure of the baby on your diaphragm may interfere with your breathing. This is not something to worry about. Continue exercising and lower your intensity, but don't overdo it. Keep hydrated—drink lots of water.

Do aerobic exercises without jumping or jarring. They're easy on your joints and back because they're all low impact. Exercising in a pool is a wonderful option.

Pelvic Floor Muscle Exercises

Prenatal exercises help you carry the baby better. Following are a series of postural exercises that work on your pelvic floor muscles, which are essential for a healthy pregnancy, delivery, and postpartum shape-up.

Your pelvic muscles are located between your legs, where they form a "floor" at the base of your pelvis, spanning a diamond from the pubic bone to the tailbone. You can feel how your pelvic floor muscles work by starting and stopping the flow of urine.

Exercise #1: Contract your pelvic floor muscles and hold for 10 seconds.

Exercise #2: Slowly contract and release, contracting your pelvic floor muscles progressively tighter to a count of five and slowly releasing to a count of five.

If you find it hard to hold for 10 seconds, begin with 3–5 seconds. Slowly increase the time as you become stronger. Begin with five repetitions of each exercise 2–3 times a day, building to 10–15 reps five to ten times a day.

Don't tense your abdomen, buttocks, and thighs when doing these exercises. Sit or stand with your legs slightly apart so you can isolate the correct area.

KEGELS

Exercises for the pelvic floor, originally developed by gynecologist Dr. A. H. Kegel, are very important during pregnancy. I do kegels all the time. When I'm in the car, every time I'm at a stoplight I remind myself to tighten up my tummy or do a kegel. They are so important now, during your pregnancy, and after delivery. Later in life, kegels can help with bladder control.

To do a kegel, simply tighten your vaginal muscles as if you are trying to stop the flow of urine. Tighten, then release. Do this ten times.

So whenever you are at a stoplight, make it a habit to tighten up your tummy or do a kegel. It takes only seconds, but it's important to do it regularly and consistently. I always do at least ten a day of each. Now, as a mom in the carpool line every day, it's a perfect time to tighten.

Dear Denise,
Do kegels really help improve your sex life?

Yes! Why do a kegel? Your vaginal muscles need exercising just as your biceps need firming. Work your vaginal muscles, pelvic tilt, and abdominal contraction. Plus, it gets you in training for pushing during delivery. Practice your kegel (contracting your vaginal canal) by comparing the exercise to rising in an elevator. Contract a little and go the first floor; contract more and go to the second floor. Keep going until you reach the top floor. Then lower slowly until you bottom out at the basement. Fully relax at the bottom.

This is the relaxed point you want to be at when you are in labor. Practice both contracting and releasing. Don't worry, you won't accidentally push your baby out! The baby is safe and secure within the womb. This is a great exercise to do every day. I personally used to do it before I went to bed. I think this exercise particularly helped me during labor and delivery. I learned how to push and relax and had some knowledge of what to expect during delivery.

Third Trimester

CHAPTER 7

Honey, You're in the Home Stretch Now

You can do it! Remember, it's only nine months of your life—and every single day counts!

This is what the last three months of pregnancy are all about. You can feel the baby kicking, reacting to noises and stimulation. The baby is also growing rapidly now, as much as half a pound per week. Congratulations! God willing, you and the baby are healthy and getting ready for the final weeks before delivery.

Your appetite is still going strong, although you might start experiencing more heartburn from time to time. Friends and family might be planning a baby shower for you. You're probably seeing your doctor every two weeks. By the ninth month your appointments will increase to once a week.

You've bought some cute maternity clothes (at least they still seem cute now—they *won't* after you've worn them a hundred times in a row), and everyone's trying to guess the sex of your baby. You're actually thinking of choices for godmother and godfather.

It's also getting harder to bend over, so now's the time to ask your husband to help tie your shoelaces or even paint your toenails!

Many pregnant women experience a surge of energy right now—cleaning out closets, rearranging furniture, even buying a new house and

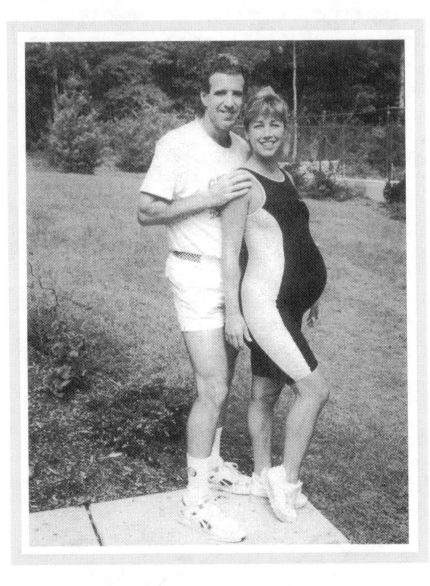

We're getting bigger, but still working out!

moving. It's called "nesting," and women have been doing it forever. Now's the time to paint the nursery (use latex only, and keep the room well ventilated) and shop for furniture and baby equipment. Just don't go overboard; pace yourself! Get help as often as possible . . . now's the best time to ask for extra help!

This is an exciting time in your pregnancy.

You should be glowing and beaming with self-confidence. You're going to be a mother very soon, and the whole world is noticing. People smile when you walk down the street. Other pregnant women feel like sisters. But sometimes people *can* go to far. Can you believe the fact that total strangers come up to you and want to feel your tummy? Some actually do.

Three months before my first daughter, Kelly, was born, I was invited by then-president George Bush to lead the nation in aerobics to celebrate the Great American Workout. I showed up at the White House in my leotard (with a tank top over it), seven months pregnant! I led the exercise routine while Bush, Arnold Schwarzenegger, and Colin Powell joined in. I'm sure they were amazed at my energy level. I was pumped!

Shortly afterward I received a signed picture from the president, with the inscription "Hey, look at that baby!"

There are so many ways in which you feel special now. People give up their seats for you. They offer you glasses of water. Your husband takes extra care of you—hopefully.

Jeff was so attentive to me, especially during my first pregnancy. He could feel the baby kicking and see the baby's heel moving across my stomach at night. It's definitely more real than it was before. He made sure he opened the door for me, carried the groceries, took out the trash, plumped up my pillows. Boy, did I play it up! I wanted to be *spoiled*. It was a time when I deserved to be put on a pedestal. Let yourself feel special!

*P*lan to bring your own pillow and your favorite pillowcase to the hospital with you. The familiar smell and feel will be cozy and comforting.

However, don't forget about your husband's self-doubts about being a good father and a good provider. Give him plenty of support and nurturing too. While this is a very exciting time, it is also quite scary.

I woke up really early during these last months, my mind racing. I was excited and probably a little anxious to know how my life was going to change. We had been married for seven years with no responsibilities but to each other and our careers.

We both wondered if we would have a boy or a girl and how our lives would be altered forever.

I NEVER WORRIED about whether I would be a good mother. I have confidence in myself and knew that nature would take over.

In my first pregnancy I did sign up early for Lamaze childbirth classes. With my second, Katie, I felt I didn't need them.

Although this is a time of great expectation, it can also be a time of worry. I remember counting the weeks, knowing that when I hit week 37, I would be able to safely deliver a healthy baby, even if it was premature. For a first-time mother, it can be scary.

> *S*tart now to practice putting the baby in and out of the car seat. Use a stuffed animal or doll, and get used to the overhead harness and the way it attaches.

I have to share the following story with you.

I had to give a lecture to executives in Captiva Island, Florida. It was the last time I could fly during my pregnancy, since you are not allowed to fly after the seventh month.

I gave my speech and later joined the corporate executives for lunch on the patio. As I sat down and started talking to them, I felt my whole bottom becoming totally wet. I was wearing a skirt and jacket, and the whole skirt was sopping. I was too afraid to tell anyone, but I thought my water had broken! I stayed in that chair until the very end of the luncheon making sure I was one of the last ones to leave. I walked with one of the women back to my hotel room. I knew she had children, and I was so worried that I asked her what I should do. She told me to call my doctor. I called him in Washington, D.C., and it felt as if I were a million miles away. He asked if I felt cramps or contractions. I didn't. In fact, I felt perfectly fine.

He said, "Are you sure the chair wasn't wet when you sat down?" I said I didn't notice it and that I didn't think they would seat me at a wet chair.

I tried to go to sleep. In the middle of the night I woke up, scared to death. I thought I felt a little cramp. I got up and looked through the telephone book and found the local hospital. I called and asked for the OB/GYN floor. I talked to a nurse and asked if they took premies. She said they didn't and that I would be flown by medevac to another hospital in Fort Myers, Florida.

I hung up the phone and sat on the bed, terrified. I had the whole plan worked out in my mind. I never went back to sleep. The next day there were no cramps and I felt fine. I later learned it *had* rained the night before the luncheon. Thank the Lord, I must have sat on a wet chair and imagined my cramps.

I know your mind is working overtime now. We *all* have anxieties and worries about what lies ahead. Here are four ways I've found to reduce your tension level:

Inhale through the nose and take three deep breaths. Exhale out the mouth. Feel your body relaxing.

Take a five-minute walk. Even a short burst of activity will calm your nerves. Exercise is a natural tranquilizer.

Close your eyes. Try to envision the most restful, peaceful scene. It may be lying in a hammock or on a float in a pool, soaking up the sun. Tense your fists, then release. Do this five times.

Listen to soothing music. It will help you relax. Sometimes if I'm feeling anxious, I put on fun music and scream out the lyrics. . . . Feel all that tension release?

As you approach labor and delivery, your worries are real. Will my baby be normal? Will I be able to handle delivery? Will I be able to breast-feed?

As each pregnancy is different, so is each labor. Remember, take all the stories you've heard or read about with a grain of salt. No two labors are alike! Every mother is different, as is every baby. Just listen to your own body and follow your instincts. Common sense is your best guide.

You can do it!

*P*ut a smile on your face. You'll get one back for sure.

We all feel vulnerable at this time in our pregnancies. No one wants to "fail." Just remember; childbirth is the most natural experience you will ever have. It's a process our bodies were designed for.

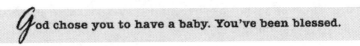

God chose you to have a baby. You've been blessed.

And don't forget that you are not alone—you will be attended to by the best medical personnel, who have years of training and practice and still manage to give every woman the impression that she is the bravest, most wonderful patient they have ever had!

MANY OF YOU are also anxious about baby care. Because we are so spread out these days, many women don't have family nearby. And because we might not live near our families (I don't), many of us have never had experience caring for a newborn. I was fortunate enough to be able to visit my sisters and friends after their babies were born. Believe me, it was the best education, watching them nurse or bottle-feed the baby and taking a turn at changing diapers.

The best advice I can give you is to just relax and enjoy the last weeks of your pregnancy, taking time out to pamper yourself a little bit.

Take five minutes and call your mother. Remember, she carried you for nine months and knows everything you're feeling.

BEAUTY TIPS FOR PREGNANCY PAMPERING

- **RESIST THE URGE TO MAKE DRASTIC CHANGES IN YOUR HAIRSTYLE OR MAKEUP. THERE ARE ENOUGH CHANGES GOING ON ALREADY.**
- **BLUNT-CUT BANGS MAKE YOUR FACE LOOK ROUNDER. FEATHER OR LAYER YOUR BANGS FOR A SOFTER LOOK.**
- **EMPHASIZE YOUR EYES AND LIPS. START USING A GOOD LIP MOISTURIZER NOW. BRING IT WITH YOU TO THE HOSPITAL.**
- **DON'T OVERDO THE BLUSHER. BRIGHT CHEEKS WILL ACCENTUATE A FULLER FACE.**

Dear Denise

I'm in my third trimester. Can I still color my hair?

There are no warnings yet on hair dye packages, so research has not shown a connection between coloring your hair and birth defects. But like any chemical that could penetrate the scalp and get into the bloodstream, hair color should be used with caution. Darker colors contain more chemicals than blond shades. My colorist recommends using foil if a pregnant woman wants to continue highlighting, and make sure there is adequate ventilation in the room. (I kept my highlights but told the colorist not to go to the root . . . just a little bit above it.)

Some medical experts also warn against getting a permanent now. Pregnancy hormones can cause hair to react to the chemicals in unusual ways, resulting in a frizzy or flat hairstyle rather than a curly look. Wait until after the baby is born to do anything complicated to your hair.

THIRD TRIMESTER HEALTH QUESTIONS

Q. *I've noticed a yellowish discharge from my breasts. Is this normal?*

A. *Yes, especially if you squeeze your breasts. This thin liquid is called* colostrum, *and I began noticing it toward my eighth month. This substance— a mixture of water, protein, and minerals—is what your baby will get for the first few days of nursing before your milk comes in. It provides antibodies and other nutrients the baby needs that protect against disease. I know it can be a little messy, but inserting a soft cotton pad into your bra will help. Not all women develop colostrum at this stage, so if you are not leaking, don't worry! It is* not *a prediction of whether you will be successful at breast-feeding.*

Q. *How can I get comfortable enough to have a good night's sleep?*

A. *Many women find it difficult to find a comfortable position as they head into their final months. You should lie on your left side to assist circulation and raise your knee to eliminate back pressure. Here's a picture of me with my propped-up pillows, which always helped me get a good night's sleep, although there were many nights when the baby was kicking all night long! They seem to get their nights and days mixed up. If you haven't gotten a good night's sleep, try to take a short nap. Rest is crucial during these final weeks, and you need to gather all your strength for labor and delivery. This*

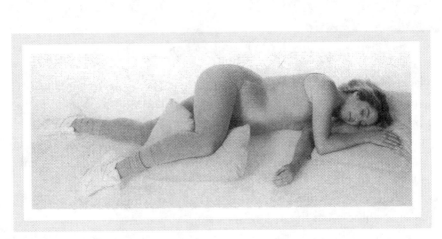

is a time when we need eight to ten hours of sleep each night to feel our best.

Exercise tip: *During the day, to help relieve the pressure the uterus puts on your diaphragm, lift your arms up and out to ease breathing and allow the rib cage to expand a bit.*

Q. *Is there any way to tell if my baby will be early or late?*

A. *No. About 80 percent of babies are born from two weeks before to two weeks after their due date. On average, premies account for 10 percent of all births. The other 10 percent arrive more than two weeks late, also known as postdate births. (My first baby was thirteen days late!) If your doctor decides, through various tests, that there are signs of a malfunctioning placenta or fetal distress, he will likely induce labor or deliver the baby by cesarean.*

Q. *How will I know when I am in labor?*

A. *Actually, some women do not know their labors have begun (lucky them!). Others know instantly. You will likely have experienced some mild, irregular contractions late in your term. These are known as Braxton Hicks contractions. These cramps are generally not painful, but they may prompt a call to your doctor. There are distinct differences between false and true labor.*

    In **true labor:** *Contractions occur at regular intervals and gradually get closer together. They will then last longer and become more intense. Most doctors recommend that you call when your contractions are five minutes apart and last forty-five seconds or more. Your cervix may be starting to dilate.*

Call your doctor if there is any doubt.

If there is any fluid rushing or leaking from your vagina, call your doctor immediately. When your water breaks or membranes rupture, the amniotic fluid escapes. Also, be aware that sometimes your water will break and come out only a little at a time.

Q. *I've heard that certain massages can be dangerous for pregnant women. Is this true?*

A. *Many doctors do not recommend therapeutic massages during pregnancy. Even massage therapists trained in treating pregnant women might not do it without a letter from your doctor. There are certain vulnerable areas in a pregnant woman's body. In particular, with women who suffer from varicose veins, massaging the inner thighs can trigger a broken blood clot, which can work its way to the heart and lungs. So save the deep, soothing massages for after delivery.*

CHAPTER 8

Give In to
Your Cravings

*N*ow you might understand all those pickle and ice cream jokes about pregnant women; food cravings are more frequent and more intense. I have a friend who craved nothing but avocados in her ninth month. Another developed a taste for anchovy paste and ate Caesar salads by the bowlful.

Of course, just as many women experience aversions to certain foods, and they can vary from one pregnancy to the next.

For every woman who craves peanut butter, there is another woman who can't stand the idea of it. But when a craving does strike, it's not a question of, "Gee, maybe I'd like a Big Mac." You want it *now!*

As Carrie Fisher once said, "Instant gratification takes too long."

Giving in to cravings isn't necessarily bad. Just because you're pregnant doesn't mean you're up for sainthood. By now you're probably sick of hearing all the "don'ts" and ready to rebel. I don't want you feeling sorry for yourself now.

Relax!

My advice has always been, if you *really* crave something, take a small bite and toss the rest away or give it to someone else. If you can't pass a fast-food restaurant without stopping for a small bag of fries, don't feel guilty. But make a deal with yourself: Limit your snack to exactly half the French fries and give the rest away. Your craving will be satisfied, but you will not consume enough fat and salt to ruin your daily regimen. If you crave cookies, take a few bites of one and then toss it. If you crave blueberry cheesecake, try blueberry yogurt. Your craving will already be satisfied by then.

Afterward, brush your teeth. Then you won't feel like eating more!

I loved Ovaltine chocolate with skim milk, hot or cold, and there's no caffeine. It always satisfied my "chocoholic" desires.

(For more suggestions, see my "crave stoppers" on page 85.)

Diet tip . . . It takes twenty minutes for your brain to register that you are "full." When you sit down to a meal, try to eat slowly. Don't rush. This will prevent you from overeating and from feeling bloated.

As your pregnancy progresses, fat stores and reserves are held in your body, especially the last two months. It's nature's way of protecting the baby and you.

Fat in your **breasts** protects the mammary glands.

A fat pad under your **kidneys** cushions the baby when you move (and also protects him if you fall—God forbid).

An extra layer of fat under your skin helps insulate you and keeps the baby warm in winter.

When fat is burned (because you haven't eaten enough good carbohydrates) a condition can result called **ketosis—acid in the blood.** So skipping meals during the last trimester to limit your weight gain is not smart. But it is a time to pay attention to your eating habits and watch your fat gram intake; in short, reduce any junk food.

With my on-the-run lifestyle, sometimes fast food is the only food available. When I'm on the road, it's not unusual for me to ask my driver to cruise past a drive-through window. And after Kelly and Katie were born, sometimes McDonald's was the only thing they wanted. I have to hand it to fast-food restaurants, though. They have recognized the need for low-fat choices and are now offering even more alternatives to fatty burgers and fries.

All it takes is knowing what to ask for. So instead of skipping a meal, know that fast food can be an acceptable alternative. Just be careful what you order.

In general, try to order a skinless grilled chicken sandwich, minus any special sauce or mayonnaise. Add your own zip with mustard, ketchup, or barbecue sauce for one-quarter the fat and calories.

Ask for a whole-wheat bun, if there is one. It contains more fiber than white bread.

Order a plain baked potato topped with low-calorie dressing, salsa, or other salad bar ingredients like shredded carrots, cucumbers, and tomatoes.

If available, order pretzels instead of fries.

Always remove any skin from chicken; it contains three-quarters of the fat.

Don't give up your favorite pizza! Just ask for it without meat and cheese. You'll be surprised how quickly you can adapt to just having plain pizza sauce with a little sprinkled Parmesan cheese for a lot less fat and calories.

Here are some of my favorite choices from popular fast-food establishments:

McDonald's

Garden salad with fat-free herb vinaigrette
(85 calories, 0 gram fat)
Single hamburger with bun (260 calories, 9 grams fat)
Grilled Chicken Deluxe Salad (120 calories, 1.5
grams fat)
Vanilla reduced-fat ice-cream cone (150 calories,
4 grams fat)

Burger King

BK broiler chicken sandwich (550 calories,
10 grams fat)
BK broiler chicken garden salad with reduced-fat
Italian dressing (200 calories, 10 grams fat)

Wendy's

Small chili (210 calories, 7 grams fat)
Grilled chicken fillet sandwich with tomato and
mustard (275 calories, 7 grams fat)
Grilled chicken Caesar salad with reduced-fat Italian
dressing (300 calories, 12 grams fat)

Roy Rogers

Roast beef sandwich, with lettuce, tomato, pickles, onions, and mustard (335 calories, 10 grams fat)

Baked potato (130 calories, 0 gram fat)

Mashed potatoes with gravy (112 calories, 0 grams fat)

Hardees

Ham sub, side salad with fat-free dressing (390 calories, 7 grams fat)

Chicken and pasta salad with low-calorie dressing (239 calories, 4 grams fat)

Arby's

Light roast chicken deluxe on multigrain bun with lettuce and tomato (276 calories, 6 grams fat)

Light roast turkey deluxe (260 calories, 7 grams fat)

Subway

Veggie Delite (237 calories, 3 grams fat)

Turkey breast (289 calories, 4 grams fat)

Subway club (312 calories, 5 grams fat)

Domino's

2 slices 12-inch cheese pizza (360 calories, 10 grams fat)

Chick-Fil-A

*Char-grilled chicken salad with light Italian dressing
(148 calories, 3.1 grams fat)*

*Char-grilled chicken sandwich (280 calories,
3 grams fat)*

Boston Market

Turkey sandwich (312 calories, 2 grams fat)

Chicken breast sandwich (422 calories, 4 grams fat)

New potatoes (129 calories, 3.5 grams fat)

Zucchini marinara (89 calories, 3.9 grams fat)

Long John Silver's

*Ocean chef salad with fat-free ranch dressing
(160 calories, 1 gram fat)*

Popeye's

Spicy and mild tenders (110 calories, 7 grams fat)

*Mashed potatoes—no gravy (100 calories,
6 grams fat)*

Jack-in-the-Box

Chicken fajita pita (280 calories, 4 grams fat)

Obviously nutrition in the last trimester is important, even if we do slip up now and then. Don't feel guilty! Sometimes all it takes is a little planning to eat healthful meals without running to the grocery store in the evening or slaving all day in the kitchen. During the last month of my pregnancy I remember being tired by the end of the day. All I wanted to do when I came home was put my feet up. For that reason it was important to at least plan what I would have for dinner and even do some of the cooking in the morning, when I had more energy.

Also, many pregnant women in their third trimester suffer from **heartburn**. There *are* some ways to help alleviate this discomfort—here are my tips:

1. Chew gum or suck candy—this can stimulate stomach acid and help digestion.
2. Try to eat slowly. Don't gulp your meal down.
3. Avoid lying down after eating.
4. Try to limit fluids with your meals (drink in between).
5. Try to eat several smaller meals during the day.
6. Avoid spicy, greasy, or fried foods.
7. Ask your doctor what types of antacids are safe to take or chew papaya enzyme which is a digestive aid.
8. Sleep with a few stacked pillows to elevate your head and shoulders.

The baby's brain is developing throughout pregnancy, and near the end of the third trimester brain cells multiply at a rapid pace. So **protein** is expecially important now. Try to eat about 70 grams each day. Refer to p. 83 to see in which foods you can find high amounts of protein.

Carbohydrates are also important now during the last weeks of pregnancy. Do not go on a low-carb diet. Carbohydrates are needed for the development of the baby's brain and nervous system. They will also help give you energy for labor. Choose the healthier ones: beans, whole-wheat grains, veggies, and fruit. Stay away from cakes and chips. Remember, choose carbs that give you the "extras" along the way.

Good fiber choices: (low calorie) grapefruit, celery, carrots, green peppers.

(Medium calorie): raisins, apricots, nuts, and seeds.

Beans are so easy to prepare and offer so much nutritional value, now that you are in the home stretch. I began cooking with lentils and found them to be a great source of protein. They can be added to prepared fat-free soups or to plain broth for a healthy treat.

Sometimes I would just marinate them in a simple vinaigrette and serve over Bibb lettuce leaves.

Be careful not to overcook dried beans. They can get mushy. I like to cook them in defatted chicken or veal stock for extra flavor, if I have some on hand. Also, I liked adding some chopped onion or a garlic clove to the broth or water.

WELL, IT'S GETTING toward the end. You're in the last trimester. Hooray! Along with increased movements of the baby, you may be experiencing more swelling and even heartburn, which can make eating uncomfortable. Try small, frequent meals, and move around after eating. Watch highly seasoned and fatty foods, and try to limit the caffeine. Although swelling is a natural part of pregnancy, you may feel better if you limit highly salted items and increase high-potassium foods (such as fruits and vegetables).

MEAL PLANS

Breakfast

Fruit smoothie—blend together:

6 ounces low-fat yogurt, fruit flavored

5-inch banana (avoid bananas if you are constipated)

½ cup frozen strawberries

4 ounces orange juice

4 ounces skim milk

1 slice toast with 1 teaspoon whipped butter and

cinnamon-sugar

Midmorning

1 grapefruit

8 ounces glass water

Lunch

A chef's salad with:

2 cups raw vegetables

¼ cup shaved turkey breast

¼ cups shredded part-skim cheese

½ cup canned garbanzo beans, rinsed

2 tablespoons vinaigrette

1 cinnamon-raisin bagel with 1 tablespoon apple butter

8 ounces flavored seltzer water

Midafternoon

1 scoop (¾ cup) frozen yogurt with frozen or fresh
   peaches
   (½ cup)

8 ounces glass water

Dinner

4-ounce chicken breast marinated in a mix of equal
   parts honey and mustard and a splash of lemon
   juice—put ¼ inch water in the bottom of the pan,
   cover with foil, and bake at 350 degrees for 30
   minutes

⅔ cup steamed rice with 1 teaspoon whipped butter

1 cup steamed green beans and mushrooms

8 ounces glass skim milk

Total

Calories: 1,926

Fat: 42 grams

Potassium: 3,685 milligrams

Sodium: 1,639 milligrams

Calcium: 1,400 milligrams

Carbohydrate 62 percent, Protein 20 percent,

Fat 18 percent

Here are a few of my favorite recipes for the third trimester.

South Austin Lentil and Avocado Salad

(Serves 4)

■

1 CUP LENTILS

½ CUP LOW-FAT SOUR CREAM

JUICE OF 1 LIME OR LEMON

1 TABLESPOON CHOPPED CILANTRO

1 TOMATO, CHOPPED

SALT AND PEPPER TO TASTE

½ CUP COOKED BLACK BEANS (CANNED)

ENDIVE OR BIBB LETTUCE LEAVES

1 RIPE AVOCADO, PEELED, PITTED, AND CUBED

Cook lentils according to package directions in water or broth. Drain.

In a bowl, whisk together the sour cream, lime or lemon juice, cilantro, tomato, and salt and pepper. Add beans and lentils, and stir. Add avocado and spoon over lettuce leaves. *Note:* Don't add the avocado unless you are going to serve the salad immediately. It will turn brown.

Sometimes I would also serve this as a healthy dip, with low-fat tortilla chips.

Texas Flank Steak

(Serves 4)

∎

1 MEDIUM TO LARGE FLANK STEAK OR LONDON BROIL
$\frac{1}{4}$ CUP KETCHUP
3 TABLESPOONS DARK BROWN SUGAR
$\frac{1}{4}$ CUP LOW-SODIUM SOY SAUCE
DASH OF WORCESTERSHIRE SAUCE
1 TEASPOON GARLIC SALT
2 TABLESPOONS A-1 STEAK SAUCE

In an airtight container, mix all the marinade ingredients. Stir well to blend. Add steak and turn once or twice to coat the meat. (I use my hands!)

Refrigerate the steak. (I usually prepare this in the morning and let it sit all day.)

Grill over hot coals, or broil, until done.

Nutmeg Sweet Potatoes

(Serves 4)

∎

Sweet potatoes are an excellent source of beta-carotene, vitamin A, and vitamin B$_6$.

$1\frac{1}{2}$ POUNDS SWEET POTATOES, PEELED AND CUT INTO
1-INCH PIECES
2 TABLESPOONS OLIVE OIL
2 TEASPOONS MINCED GARLIC (OPTIONAL)
NUTMEG

Preheat oven to 450 degrees.

In a large pot of boiling water, add the potatoes and cook until just tender, five minutes or so. Drain the potatoes and immediately plunge them into a bowl of ice water to stop the cooking process. Drain again and blot dry with a paper towel.

Place the potatoes in a large roasting pan and add oil and garlic. Turn to coat all sides and place in oven, turning two or three times until the potatoes are nicely browned, about fifteen minutes. Place in serving dish and sprinkle a bit of nutmeg on top.

Pasta with Basil, Tomato, and Olives

(Serves 4)

■

This dish should be made in the morning and allowed to marinate all day, or at least for several hours.

½ CUP OLIVE OIL
½ CUP SHREDDED FRESH BASIL
4 RIPE TOMATOES, SEEDED AND CHOPPED
1 CLOVE GARLIC, PEELED AND FINELY MINCED
8 LARGE BLACK OLIVES, PITTED AND HALVED
SALT AND FRESHLY GROUND PEPPER
PASTA: 1 POUND LINGUINE, THIN SPAGHETTI,
OR SPAGHETTI

In a medium-size mixing bowl, stir together the olive oil, basil, tomatoes, garlic, and olives until well blended. Cover with plastic wrap and let sit in a cool place (or in the summer put it in the refrigerator). I usually make this in the morning, it's so easy.

Cook pasta according to package directions. Drain. Put pasta back into the pot and add the tomato-basil mixture. Toss well and serve with pinch of fresh basil as garnish.

Note: Sometimes I like to add a little cheese, if I happen to have some on hand. Shredded low-fat mozzarella adds a creamy texture to the sauce, or try a little crumbled goat cheese.

This pasta is excellent served hot or cold.

Food tip . . . Keep healthy snacks in your desk, purse, or car. I used to keep a stash of cheese-and-cracker snack packs, snack-size canned tuna, fat-free pretzel sticks, and rice cakes in the glove compartment for minimeals on the go. It will sometimes take the place of a fast-food stop.

During pregnancy your immune system is suppressed, making you more vulnerable to illness caused by bacteria and parasites. Err on the side of caution when handling food. Vomiting and/or diarrhea will dehydrate you and can increase the risk of pre-term labor.

- **BE SURE TO COOK RED MEAT AND POULTRY UNTIL THEY ARE DONE. WHEN YOU ARE EATING OUT, IT'S WISE DURING PREGNANCY TO ASK FOR MEDIUM-WELL TO WELL-DONE MEAT.**
- **COOK EGGS UNTIL THE WHITES AND YOLKS ARE FIRM.**
- **EAT ONLY COOKED SEAFOOD. AVOID SUSHI AND SASHIMI.**
- **AVOID FOODS WITH RAW EGGS (NO MORE COOKIE DOUGH).**

Dear Denise

I've just been diagnosed with diabetes and I'm in my ninth month of pregnancy. How should I change my diet?

Hormonal changes can often trigger a mild case of diabetes in pregnant women. This is temporary. Gestational diabetes strikes about 3 percent of mothers and usually disappears after delivery. You will be asked to take a glucose tolerance test early in your third trimester. If diabetes is confirmed, you will probably be given a special diet and exercise plan by your doctor, depending on your blood sugar. In some cases insulin will be prescribed.

Women at risk for gestational diabetes are those with a family history of it, overweight women, and older mothers.

A new study from the University of Southern California School of Medicine shows that among women with pregnancy-related diabetes, those who have a second baby have three times the risk of developing adult-onset diabetes (also known as *type II diabetes*) later in life.

The best way to protect yourself is to keep your weight under control. For every ten pounds a mother gains after pregnancy, her chances of getting type II diabetes doubles.

Q. *Are herbal teas safe to drink during pregnancy?*

A. *Not all herbal teas are alike. Some are not safe for pregnant women, as they may act as laxatives or react as stimulants; both may cause uterine contractions. If there is a question, ask your doctor first. Many advise that only chamomile, ginger, and raspberry teas be consumed by pregnant women. Be sure to check with your doctor, just to be sure.*

Q. *How can I control a mild case of high blood pressure with diet?*

A. *Many pregnant women experience a slight increase in blood pressure during pregnancy, which in most cases is harmless. If high blood pressure is accompanied by swelling due to water retention and sudden weight gain (more than two pounds a week in the third trimester), see your doctor. This could signal the beginning of* **preeclampsia,** *a dangerous condition.*

But for women with a mild case of hypertension, a low-sodium diet is recommended. That means giving up pretzels, potato chips, tuna salad sandwiches, olives, soy sauce, and other salty foods. And remember to read the labels on fat-free or low-fat foods. Often they contain high amounts of sodium to make up for the lack of natural taste. Also, aquatic exercise and immersion in pools have been proven to reduce swelling.

Q. *I work in an office and have a working lunch almost every day. Is there any way to avoid heavy restaurant meals?*

A. *Yes! Toward the end of my first pregnancy I was still taking the train to New York for business meetings and often ended up with associates for lunch. Because restaurant portions tend to be large, I always asked for half orders. And salad dressing should always be ordered "on the side." That way you can control the amount you want. Often I just dipped my lettuce into the dressing. You'll eat less and still enjoy the taste.*

Here are other tips for restaurant dining:

- **ALWAYS CHOOSE CLEAR OR BROTH-BASED SOUPS OVER CREAMED ONES.**
- **ORDER A WHEAT ROLL OVER WHITE. IT CONTAINS MORE FIBER.**
- **LOOK FOR LOW-FAT, HIGH-PROTEIN MAIN COURSES SUCH AS BROILED CHICKEN OR FISH. POACHED IS EVEN BETTER. MANY CHEFS WILL ACCOMMODATE YOUR REQUEST. DON'T BE AFRAID TO ASK!**

- ASK TO SUBSTITUTE A SECOND VEGETABLE FOR THE STARCH SIDE DISH.
- IF YOU'RE CRAVING THAT CHOCOLATE MOUSSE FOR DESSERT, TAKE ONE BITE AND GIVE THE REST TO YOUR LUNCH MATES. YOU WILL SATISFY THE CRAVING WITHOUT ALL THE CALORIES.
- DRINK PLENTY OF WATER. IT WILL FILL YOU UP.

CHAPTER 9

You Can Do It! Exercises for the Third Trimester

Keeping fit right now is important for you and your baby. This is the time to prepare yourself for labor and delivery and insure a speedy recovery—to bounce right back into shape, even better than before! Follow this simple ten-minute exercise routine every day. I did it with both my pregnancies. If you don't feel you can, try for three days a week. Remember, there is no need to push yourself. Listen to your body!

Warm-up

Using a chair for balance, stand with legs apart, back straight, and toes turned out. Slowly lower body until knees are over ankles (don't go beyond the toes), then squeeze buttocks as you lift. Lower and lift for 1 minute.

REPEAT 2 sets of 8–10 reps each.

BENEFITS: Thighs (quadriceps), hamstrings, gluteals.

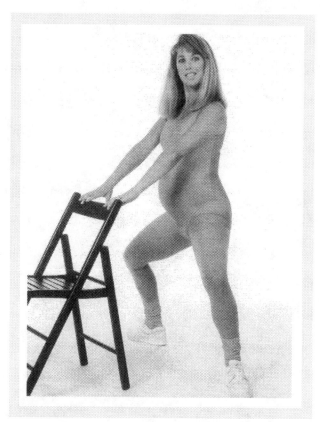

Saddlebag Slimmer

Stand with your feet together, your hands on the back of a chair for balance. Your back should be straight and your abs tight. With your foot flexed, slowly lift your right leg out to your side, then lower the leg. Be sure to keep your back straight. The movement should be slow and controlled. Repeat. When you have finished your two sets with the right leg, repeat the exercise on the left leg.

REPEAT 2 sets of 8–12 lifts each.

BENEFITS: Outer hip and thigh (abductors).

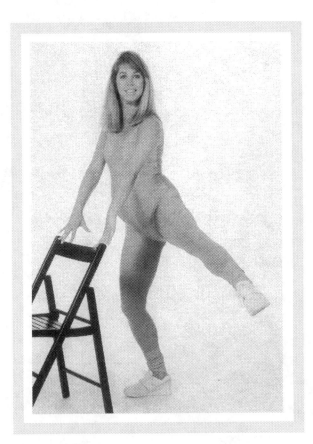

Supported Lunge

·

Start with one foot in front of the other as though you are taking a giant step. (A chair can be used for balance.)

Lower yourself, bending both knees, but make sure your knee stays in line with your ankle. Try not to bang your back knee on the floor. Your weight should be on your back toes and on your front heel.

Straighten legs until you are standing, and then lower yourself again.

REPEAT for 16–24 reps. Then repeat with opposite leg.

BENEFITS: Works the entire leg.

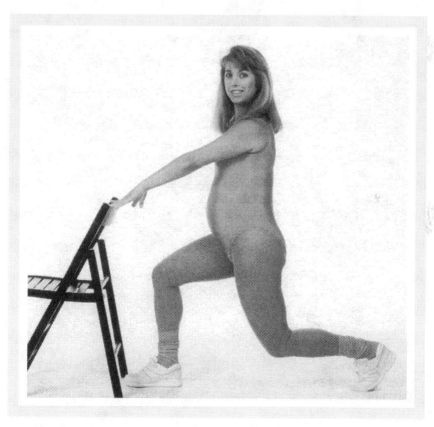

Buttocks Lift

Extend right leg. Hold for ten seconds, squeezing buns. Relax and repeat with the other leg. Contract the abs and be sure not to arch the lower back.

REPEAT 2 sets of 8–12 reps.

BENEFITS: Firms and tightens the tush.

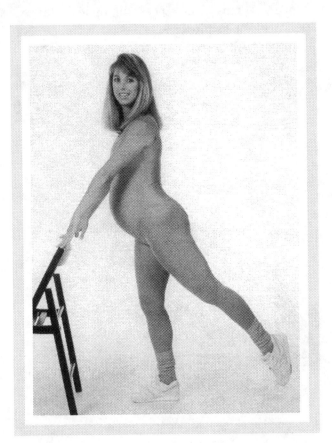

Back of Thigh Firmer

Stand up nice and tall, with your back straight and abs tight. Hold the chair for balance. Bend your right leg, keeping your foot flexed, and squeeze your buttocks. Your heel should be toward your rear end. Pulse the heel up 8–12 reps. Relax and switch legs.

REPEAT 2 sets of 8–12 reps.

BENEFITS: Firms and tightens the backs of thighs.

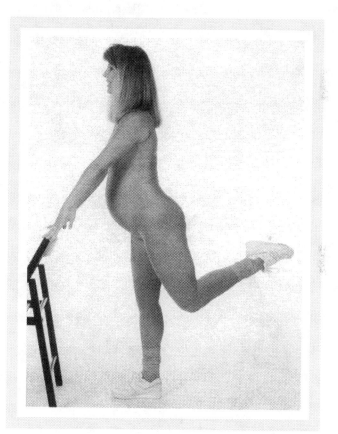

Baby Squat

Stand with your legs apart, holding on to a chair for support. Your feet should be a little wider than your hips. Your back should be straight and your abs tight. Place your hands on your hips. Bend your knees and begin to squat. Feel as though you're sitting back, with your body weight through your heels. Hips should move behind your heels, as though you're lowering yourself into a chair. As you stand back up, exhale and squeeze your buttocks.

REPEAT 2 sets of 8–12 reps each. Rest 15 seconds between sets.

BENEFITS: Thighs (quadriceps), buttocks (gluteals), hamstrings.

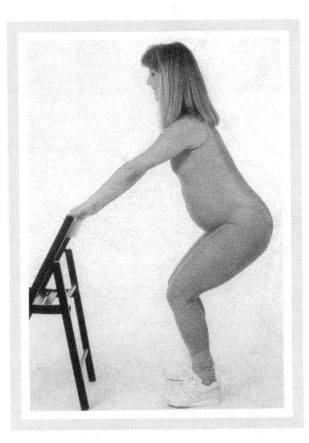

Lower Body Firmer

Get on your knees and place your arms on top of a chair for support. (This will take the pressure off your wrists and your back.) Lift your right leg and slowly lower. Do not arch the back. "Squeeze" your buttocks.

REPEAT 8–12 reps each leg.

BENEFITS: Tones and firms lower body. Great for your "rear view."

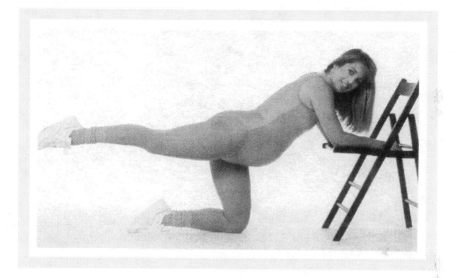

Waist Side Toner

•

This is a basic situp, done on your side. With one arm stretched out, exhale as you lift your opposite shoulder blade off the floor.

REPEAT 8–12 crunches on each side.

BENEFITS: Strengthens lateral abdominal muscles, and even some back muscles.

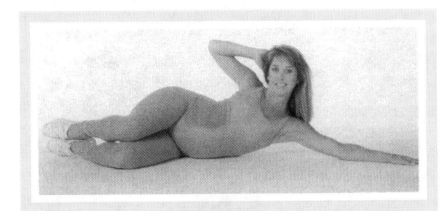

Tummy Tucks

Sit on the floor with your knees bent. Place your hand underneath your lower thigh to support your back. Slowly roll back, contracting your abdominals. Think of your muscles hugging the baby. Inhale and then exhale as you tighten abs.

A variation of this exercise is shown, with your body weight resting on your knuckles. Roll and contract your abdominals.

REPEAT 2 sets of 8–12 reps.

BENEFITS: Tightens abdominals, stretches lower back.

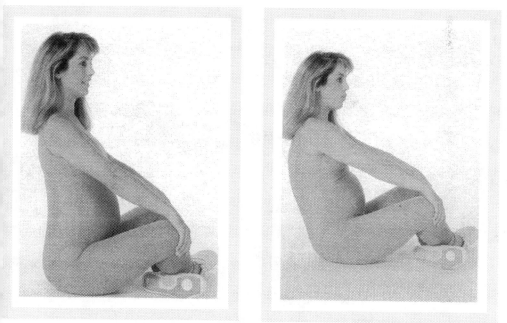

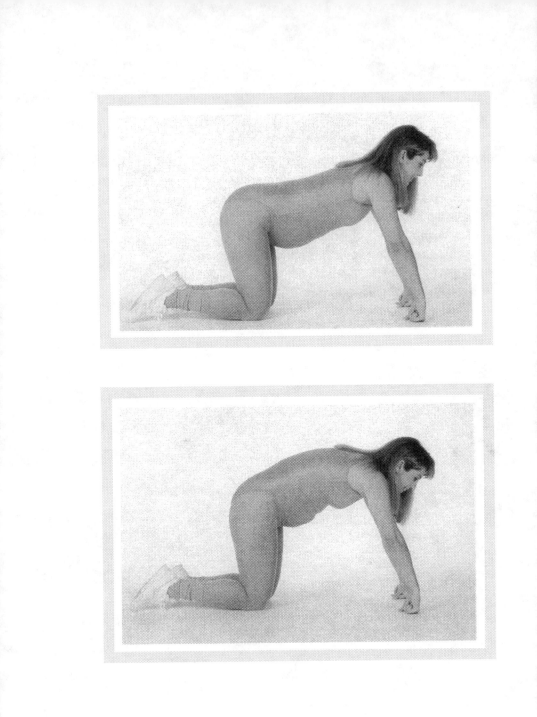

Upper Back Strengthener

Stand with your legs apart, knees slightly bent, and your back straight. Extend one arm and reach reach reach out straight ahead and then pull back, as if you are rowing a boat.

REPEAT 2 sets of 8–12 reps each per arm. Rest 15 seconds between sets.

BENEFITS: Upper back (latissimus dorsi, rhomboid), back of shoulders (posterior deltoid). Both strengthens and stretches.

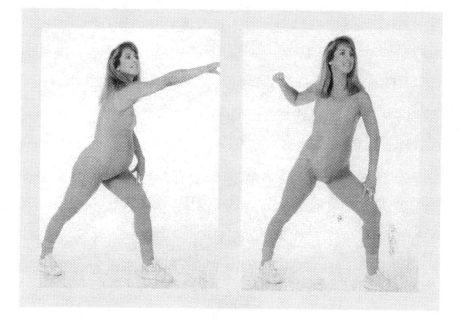

Posture Boost

•

This is an instant way to improve your posture. Pregnancy often makes us feel round shouldered and slouchy, because of the weight of your breasts and the weight of the baby. This exercise opens up the chest and increases flexibility, circulation, and oxygen flow.

Place both hands behind your head. Inhale. Hold for 3–4 seconds and release, exhaling slowly.

REPEAT 2 sets of 8–12 counts.

BENEFITS: Elongates the spine; posture perfect! Stretches the chest muscles and strengthens the upper back.

And don't forget the stretches after a workout!

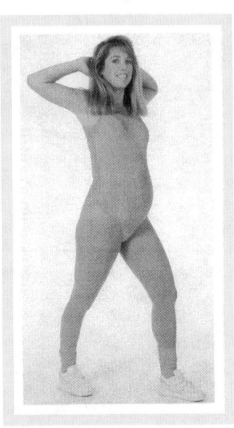

Supportive Calf Stretch

.

Stand with your hands against the wall at shoulder level, one foot forward and one foot back. Or you can stand against a chair for support.

Lean forward, bending the elbows slightly and keeping your back leg straight with your foot flat on the floor. Make sure both your feet are pointing forward. Hold for 20 seconds.

REPEAT 3 times with each leg.

BENEFITS: Stretches muscles in the back of the lower leg.

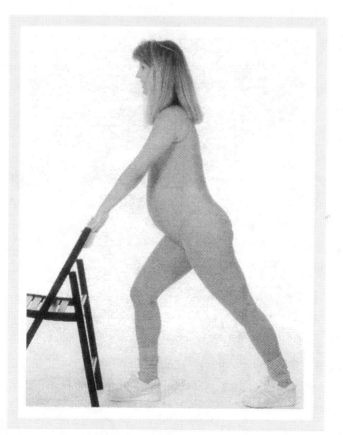

Supported Quad Stretch

Using a chair for support, place one hand on the chair and lift the opposite leg into your free hand. Hold the foot and gently pull your heel toward your buttocks. Hold for 15 seconds. Feel the stretch in the front of your thighs.

REPEAT 3 times with each leg.

BENEFITS: Flexible thighs will make walking easier.

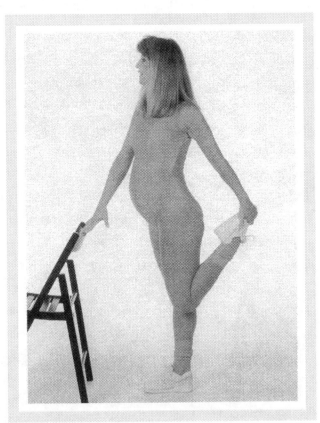

Supported Back Stretch

Using a chair for balance, get on your knees and reach your hands forward. Support your hands on the chair. Feel your shoulders and body stretch. Release and repeat.

REPEAT 3 times.

BENEFITS: To stretch your upper and lower back. This is excellent for relieving lower back pain and improving posture.

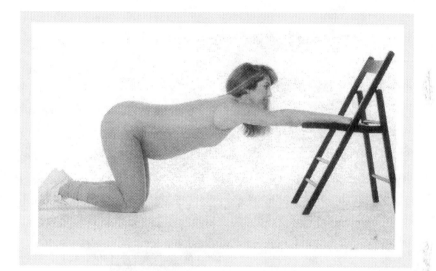

No More Slouching Shoulders

Sit cross-legged, with your hands behind your head. Feel the chest opening up. This stretch elongates the body and improves your posture. Hold stretch for 15 seconds, then relax.

REPEAT 3 times.

BENEFITS: No more slouching!

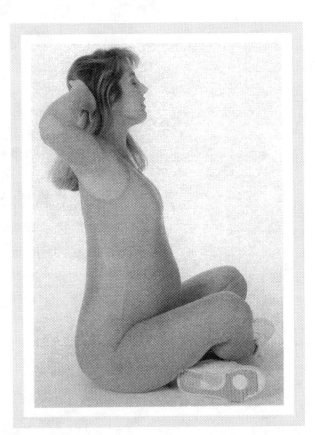

Yoga Stretch

Sit cross-legged, with your spine erect, your hands clasped behind your back. Lift your arms up while squeezing your shoulder blades back down and together. Hold for ten seconds and release.

REPEAT 3 times.

BENEFITS: This is excellent for stretching your chest muscles and straightening rounded shoulders.

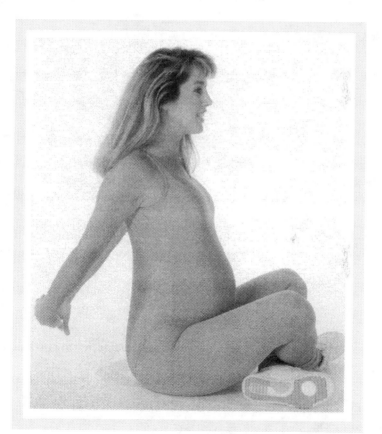

Pregnancy puts pressure on your back. You can protect your back from the extra weight by always thinking, **Perfect posture!**

1. Balance your weight around the center of gravity in your lower spine and pelvis.
2. Remember to hold your head erect, without pushing the chin forward.
3. Always keep your shoulders back and down.
4. Maintain the normal curves of your back. Stretching exercises will help.
5. Change your position often. Don't wait until your back is aching.
6. Relax. Take deep breaths. This will force chest upward.
7. Don't ever stand with your knees locked. Keep your joints loose.

The exercises I've shown you are excellent ways to tone and stretch safely, and ideally you should accompany these with your favorite aerobic activity. It could be three days a week of walking at least twenty minutes, preferably thirty to forty minutes, at a low to moderate pace, or continuing to use the stair machine or stationary bike. Whatever your body is used to.

Swimming is one of the best exercises at this point, and many women now trade in their other activities for swimming or aquatic exercise classes.

Biking is still an excellent cardiovascular workout. Many doctors recommend pregnant women give up road biking in the final months of their pregnancies. I switched to a stationary bike, just to be safe. But I know many women don't want to give it up. Research shows that moderate bicycling (thirty minutes three to four times a week) is safe for pregnant women and their babies. However, in the last trimester the risk of falling off an outdoor bike outweighs the benefits. Shift to indoor cycling or swimming.

Because of your changing center of gravity and pregnancy hormones, you are more prone to falls now. As with any exercise, if you feel any pain or shortness of breath, stop.

Did you know . . . the placentas of active, pregnant women are larger and more efficient in supplying the fetus with oxygen than those of nonactive women?

Many of you ask me exactly how many calories you burn when you exercise. The average person, while running or walking at a brisk pace, burns about one hundred calories a mile. Of course, the three-mile walk will take longer than the three-mile run, but you still burn the same number of calories.

Dear Denise

I feel so overheated all the time. Is this normal during pregnancy?

Pregnancy raises your basal metabolic rate about 20 percent, making you feel warmer—even in winter. You might notice that you perspire more or even experience "night sweats." I always tell women to dress in layers and to drink lots of liquids to keep hydrated.

ENDORPHINS

Exercise is the single best antidote to stress in everyday life. It is known to stimulate the release of **endorphins**, a natural antidepressant.

All forms of exercise prompt you to use muscles in a different way, which forces oxygen-rich blood to flow through your body, increasing your alertness and improving your mood. Exercise can result in a "natural high." For pregnant women this is especially important, since the last few weeks before delivery can be stressful.

Try to exercise in the morning, if possible. Exercise gives you energy. And you need energy during the day, not at night.

Dear Denise

I live in a humid climate. Is it safe to exercise while I'm pregnant? I'm afraid of getting overheated.

The key here is to use common sense.

Any exercise that raises your temperature more than two degrees should be avoided. Since I lived in Washington, D.C., during both my pregnancies, I endured the hot, sticky, hair-frizzing, steamy summers. Because of the humidity, I made sure to exercise only in the early morning or in the evening when the temperature cooled down. On many days I chose to stay indoors and walk on the treadmill or do step aerobics on a four-inch level step. I was working my hips, thighs, and buttocks while keeping up my cardiovascular activity. Be careful with step aerobics after the sixth month. If you look down and can't see the step over your belly, be careful. It's not worth a fall.

I did take the bounce and any complicated choreography out of my aerobic routine and modified it to very basic movements. But I didn't sacrifice anything by taking it down to the basics, and I still maintained my fitness level at this point in my pregnancy.

This was when I really tried to exercise every day.

I even did a thirty-minute walk the day I delivered my second daughter, Katie. With my first child, Kelly, I did aerobics the day I delivered. I was a little breathless—but that's normal with such a big tummy. I just took my time and tried to make my movements slow and steady.

TAKE THE TALK TEST

If you feel out of breath, try to say a sentence.

If you can't finish the sentence, you're probably pushing yourself too hard.

If you finish the sentence easily, pick up your pace slightly.

SO NOW IS *not* the time to stop.

Pregnancy should not be a state of confinement. It's a special time. Get out and enjoy life and move, move, move. Pregnancy is a miraculous journey. When you're feeling tired and uncomfortable and overwhelmed, think of this wonderful baby that is developing life inside you.

You can do it! You—and your baby—are worth it!

Dear Denise

Is it common to get hemorrhoids during pregnancy?

Yes. Some studies show that as much as 50 percent of all pregnant women will experience **hemorrhoids.** These are commonly known as varicose veins of the rectum, and become swollen and enlarged owing to constipation and increased pressure from the uterus. Toward the end of both my pregnancies I did get hemorrhoids, which resulted in my changing my daily workout. I stopped doing squats or lunges; they were too painful. Walking felt a little easier.

I also ate more fruits; my friends would laugh at me every day when I showed up at the pool with my little bag of fruit: apple, cantaloupe, grapes, or cubes of watermelon.

I also tried adding more fiber to my diet, which helped. Drinking lots of water is essential. You can also help prevent hemorrhoids by avoiding long hours of sitting or standing, taking a warm sitz bath, and doing your kegels. Try exercising in the water if land aerobics gets too uncomfortable. If you have hemorrhoids accompanied by rectal bleeding, tell your doctor.

Note: Don't use any topical medications without first checking with your doctor.

Dear Denise

I'm in my third trimester and I have chronic back pain. Is there any exercise I can do that might help?

Yes. If you are experiencing more pressure on your lower spine, one way to solve that is by using a stationary, recumbent bicycle. (It has a backrest.) Your heart rate is still up, but you're not putting pressure on your lower body.

THIRD TRIMESTER EXERCISE QUESTIONS

Q. *What is the best way physically to get ready for delivery?*
A. *Overall fitness is the key. Regular exercise will give you the stamina and strength you will need to go through labor. My abdominal exercises will help you understand how your muscles can contract and release. Once you become aware of this sensation, it will be second nature. Maintaining strong pelvic floor muscles will also help.*

Practice your abdominals (standing up), and do your kegels several times a day. Remember, when you go into labor, each experience is different. There are circumstances you cannot control, no matter how fit you are.

Q. *Will regular exercise really help shorten my labor?*

A. *Yes. Studies support this! Under normal conditions, regular exercise can shorten the amount of time a woman will be in labor because she will have more strength and stamina and a positive mental attitude. Strong abdominals will help you push more effectively. Doing your kegels will help the muscles stretch during delivery.*

Q. *Is there any way to prevent having an episiotomy?*

A. *Most doctors cannot predict who will need this procedure, which involves cutting the perineum to enlarge the opening the baby will pass through. Seventy percent of all women in North America have episiotomies. Research has shown that many runners and walkers have episiotomies. Since toned muscles are healthier and would be able to stretch more, doing kegels may help prevent an episiotomy. Hot or warm compresses may work sometimes. Also, ask your delivery nurse to try massaging your perineal area during labor. This truly helped me avoid tearing or having an episiotomy. More than anything, healthy tissue repairs more quickly. So, do your kegels and hope your doctor doesn't have a golf game!*

Q. *Will being fit during pregnancy reduce my chances of having a cesarean?*

A. *Yes. Unfortunately, my sister was disappointed to have a cesarean, since she felt she did everything right to prepare for a natural delivery. She ate right and exercised until the last day of her term. Afterward she felt robbed of the natural birth experience, but we kept telling her, "It's okay. God gave you a healthy baby."*

There is no way to predict whether you will be able to deliver your baby naturally. Twenty-three percent of pregnant women have C-sections. But exercise can reduce your chances of a C-section by 24 percent. However, my sister since has had three C-sections, and all three kids are great!

God willing, you will have a healthy baby no matter how it comes out.

Q. *I'm in my last month and my doctor told me to stop exercising. I'm worried that I won't be strong enough for labor.*

A. *If your doctor tells you, for whatever reason, to ease up on your exercise routine, don't feel bad. You will still be stronger and more fit than if you* didn't exercise at all for the last nine months. The last weeks of no activity won't undo all the good you have already done your body—and your baby! Being well rested will help you during labor, delivery, and recovery.

Q. *Can exercise cause uterine contractions?*

A. *The uterus contracts when it experiences any excess stress. In most cases these contractions are not noticeable, except to the touch. Learn to recognize these contractions by placing the fingers just below the diaphragm. A uterine contraction will feel hard to the touch. Your obstetrician can help you identify what this feels like. Although these contractions are not harmful, they may indicate that your exercise is too strenuous and you should modify your activity. Contractions may also start just because you became dehydrated during exercise. Don't forget your eight glasses of water! Keep hydrated, and please do everything in moderation. . . .* Listen to your body.

Q. *Should I stop exercising if I feel increased pressure on my pelvis and abdomen?*

A. *You might want to continue to modify the intensity of your exercise routine (make it easier) as you go into the home stretch. You'll have less oxygen available during your aerobic workout, so it might be best to switch to a slow twenty-minute walk. That's better than nothing at all! Remember, aquatic exercise and swimming are the best activities now because they put almost no pressure on your pelvis.*

Forgo the lunges and squats. They're great leg exercises, but if you have pressure, you can continue to keep your legs toned and firm by lying on your side and doing leg lifts. You can still use weights in the last weeks of your pregnancy to tone your upper body. But if you have pressure on the pelvic area, do this in a seated position, on a chair or weight bench, or sitting on the floor. Give yourself plenty of time twenty-four to forty-eight hours between each weight-training session to recover.

If you are using a weight machine at the gym, bring it down a notch. (You might already have noticed that some of the machines simply won't accommodate you in your condition.) Don't be surprised to find that you must modify your weight lifting toward the end of your pregnancy. Your center of gravity has shifted, making it more tricky to perform some of your regular exercises. Make sure to support yourself so that you feel comfortable with each movement.

If you are getting overtired, you're doing too much. Take it easy.

Q. *Can exercise help reduce swelling in pregnant women?*

A. *Exercise can reduce swelling by increasing circulation. Many women retain fluids late in their pregnancies, and almost 75 percent develop a mild form of edema (pregnancy-associated water retention) in the last weeks of their pregnancies. It's particularly common in warm weather. To ease the discomfort in ankles and legs, elevate your legs, lie on your side, get in a pool and/or make sure you are drinking plenty of water.*

Note: This is an important time to watch your salt intake. Stay away from foods high in sodium, which increase fluid retention. At the grocery store, read the labels! Many times salt is increased in low-fat food to add flavor. Also be aware that mineral water, while high in calcium, can also be high in sodium.

Buy a pair of shoes half a size larger than you normally would. Support hose is also helpful.

Q. *My doctor has recommended full bed rest for the last three weeks of my pregnancy. Is there any way I can keep my spirits up?*

A. *Bed rest should certainly be taken seriously, for your sake and the sake of your baby. But you can ask your doctor if you can do some isometric exercises. If you can, flip to the next chapter and follow the postbirth bed rest program. Also take advantage of my circulatory exercises, which will help relax you.*

Ask your husband to rub your shoulders and feet. Invest in some moisturizing creams. Pamper yourself!

You might also turn back to the first trimester section of this book and try to incorporate some of my modified stretching routines. But as always, ask your doctor first.

And don't worry! It's a small sacrifice for such a lasting reward.

LAST SOOTHING WORDS OF ADVICE BEFORE DELIVERY

- **YOU WILL GET TO THE HOSPITAL ON TIME. YOUR HUSBAND MIGHT BE A LITTLE PANICKY RIGHT NOW AND HAVING NIGHTMARES ABOUT NOT MAKING IT ON TIME. REASSURE HIM THAT BABIES, ESPECIALLY THE FIRST, TAKE HOURS TO ARRIVE.**
- **YOU WILL NOT BE ALONE.**
- **CHILDBIRTH IS A NATURAL PROCESS.**
- **YOU HAVE NOTHING TO BE AFRAID OF.**

- **YOU ARE STRONG AND HEALTHY, AND SO IS YOUR BABY.**
- **YOUR HUSBAND WILL NOT FAINT. HE WILL BE FAR TOO BUSY.**
- **REMIND YOURSELF HOW EXCITED YOU WERE WHEN YOU LEARNED YOU WERE FIRST PREGNANT AND HOW LUCKY YOU ARE! YOU CAN DO IT!**
- **THE GOOD TIMES ARE JUST BEGINNING. YOUR CHILD WILL GIVE BACK TO YOU MORE THAN YOU'LL EVER REALIZE.**

MY PERSONAL LABOR AND DELIVERY STORIES

With Kelly, my first daughter, I was thirteen days late.

Every morning I woke up thinking, Today is *the* day. But nothing was happening. So I can relate if you are reading this and wondering how much longer you have to wait. But don't worry. The baby does come out, sooner or later.

So many of my friends told me what to do to get labor going. One was sex (yeah, sure!), one was walking briskly (I had already been doing that), and one was spicy foods. Jeff remembers my wanting to eat pizza every night straight for about a week before the baby was born. (That didn't work, either, and I only gained extra fat.)

Finally, on the thirteenth day after my due date, I worked out doing step aerobics for twenty minutes, and that night I started to feel some labor pains. I called my doctor, and he said to time them. When they were eight minutes apart, he told me to go to the hospital. I crouched down and rocked my hips from side to side because I was experiencing back labor. Jeff got behind me and rubbed my lower back.

We drove to the hospital (I made Jeff stop and get me a bagel and a banana, because I was hungry and felt I needed the energy) and I was dilated to only one centimeter. The nurses encouraged me to go into town and take a walk for a good hour. Here I am, in Georgetown, on a lively summer evening at nine P.M. with people jamming the sidewalks, and I was up and down those streets for an hour, leaning over every so often with terrible cramps. Everyone looked at me, and a few even said, "Shouldn't you be going to the hospital? It's right down the street." Then the pains got worse, and I started to throw up on the sidewalk. Jeff said, "That's it. We're going back. I'm too nervous."

I got back to the hospital. They checked me again: I was at four centimeters. This is usually the perfect time to give an epidural. However, by the time they admitted me they said I was too far along for the epidural.

So I did it drug-free, but don't think it was my choice! Honey, nobody gave me a medal for doing it that way. It took all night to dilate fully, and Kelly was born at ten A.M. the next day. It took two hours to push her out. (Boy, did she have a pointy head!) But don't worry. The baby's head is so soft to allow it to pass through the birth canal, and it took shape quickly, after a day or two.

I was lucky to have a normal labor and delivery, with no complications. I have to believe that because I had exercised and was in good shape, I had enough stamina to go through it and recover quickly. I believe that you can have a similar experience, and everything you have done for yourself in the previous months will pay off. I promise! Remember, you can do it!

FIRST DELIVERY: twelve hours

KELLY AUSTIN: six pounds, nine ounces
19½ inches long

With my second daughter, my experience was different.

First of all, she was born on her due date. Thank God I got to the hospital on time! That day I took a forty-five-minute walk, strolling Kelly, and I let Jeff play in a local tennis tournament. I felt great. Jeff came home at six P.M., and I was getting ready to go the tennis tournament party and told him I felt a little cramp, but I was fine. The babysitter came for Kelly. She got there, and I was leaning over every twenty minutes, but it wasn't bad. Jeff said, "Are you sure you want to go to this party? We don't have to go." I said, "No. I feel fine. If I have to lean over and take deep breaths, I will." But I truly didn't think this was labor.

We were driving to the party around eight P.M. and I said, "Jeff, the pain's getting worse." He said, "Let's just go to the hospital."

We got there, and a young nurse looked at me and said, "Oh no, not another woman in labor! Well, it is a full moon tonight, and we'll have to put you in this recovery room until there's a labor room available."

When she checked my cervix, I was dilated to only one centimeter, she said. She told me I was probably dehydrated. I told her I had drunk over ten glasses of water that day. So she left to arrange an ultrasound for me. I didn't see her again for another thirty minutes. By that time I was crying and throwing up. We were all by ourselves in that little room. I knew something was wrong because of the pain, and I needed help. Jeff went out into the hall and grabbed a nurse. She said, "Oh, my God, the baby's here!"

Within a minute a doctor was pulled in from another labor room and a full delivery team came. They were great, and so was Jeff. She was born right there on the little twin-size recovery bed. This was my second delivery, and it's not uncommon to have a shorter delivery, but not that short. It all happened so quickly, my name wasn't even on the maternity board. I hadn't been admitted to Georgetown Hospital, and my poor doctor wasn't even there. They thought at first they were just going to send me home. Little did we know that Katie would arrive so fast. Thank God there were no complications and she was so healthy. We were fortunate, but it was so sudden. I often think *if* I did ever have a third baby, I'd have to move right next the hospital to get there on time! As you can tell, I had a quick delivery with Katie. I went from walking into that hospital to holding my baby in my arms all within less than an hour!

Second Delivery	**forty-five minutes**
Katie Austin	**six pounds, four ounces**
	19½ inches long

*B*eing a mom is a labor of love.

PEP TALK

Remember, labor is called labor for a good reason. If you enter it with strong, muscular tone and control, there is no question you will be able to function better. If you have stamina, you will be able to withstand the physical workout and recover quickly and more easily and not be totally drained. I honestly felt pretty good after both deliveries. You will tell your baby's birth story so many times, and it's a wonderful feeling of accomplishment. It's like finishing a marathon, crossing the finish line with your baby, and winning first prize!

My prayers are with you. Good luck. I know you will have the courage to do it.

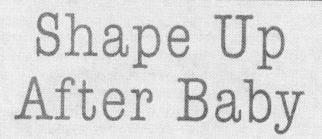

Part Four

Shape Up After Baby

CHAPTER 10

You're a Mom Now!

*Y*ou're a mom now! Congratulations!

Isn't it unbelievable? It's God's miracle. Life *is* beautiful.

Your precious little baby is finally here, and now it's time to get yourself back to feeling and looking healthy and fit.

No one can really prepare you for the postpartum experience. The incredible high of childbirth can be followed by a period of fatigue and emotional unrest. If you've had a C-section, or if your labor and delivery were especially complicated, you might be feeling more tired.

Remember, no one has the birth experience they plan for, and everyone's is different.

It's not easy to recover from childbirth with a snap of your fingers, and you might be feeling a little bit down. But just do the best you can, and don't forget . . . this time will pass very quickly, I *promise.*

Throughout your pregnancy we focused on nutrition, exercise, and having a healthy baby. But now that your little bundle of joy has arrived, there is so much to do for the baby that you might not take time to recover yourself. And now is when you need help. Hopefully your husband has already begun to pitch in, or your mother or mother-in-law has arrived to stay with you, not to mention friends who are offering to bring you dinners (and always say yes). And some of you may be worried about when to return to work, on top of everything else.

Don't even think about all that now.

My best advice during those first few weeks after the baby is born is to try to rest. Sleep when your baby sleeps. I know if you have other children it's hard, but you need your strength. It's also the time to truly enjoy your baby. Your newborn becomes an infant, and an infant becomes a toddler in a very short time!

Every time I smell a newborn, I instantly remember holding Kelly, and Katie, nursing them and feeling the joy of their warm little bodies against mine. Their baby blankets, so soft and powdery. Their slippery bodies as you give them their first bath. Toweling them and swaddling them. They smell so wonderful! Innocent and milky. I honestly think those first few weeks make you completely forget any discomfort you might have had, and all you know is unconditional love.

Enjoy . . . enjoy.

Naturally you will have many questions for your doctor, and now that you are a new mother you should not be afraid to call for advice. Fortunately I have a great OB/GYN, Dr. Joseph W. Giere, whom I often turned to. I want to share with you an interview we did for my *Pregnancy Plus* video that answers some of your basic questions about recovering from childbirth.

Q. *When should a woman begin exercising after giving birth?*
A. *Assuming you've had a normal delivery, I'd have you exercising the day after delivery. Begin with exercises in bed, doing simple leg stretches. Pay particular attention to the pelvic floor exercise and then slowly and*

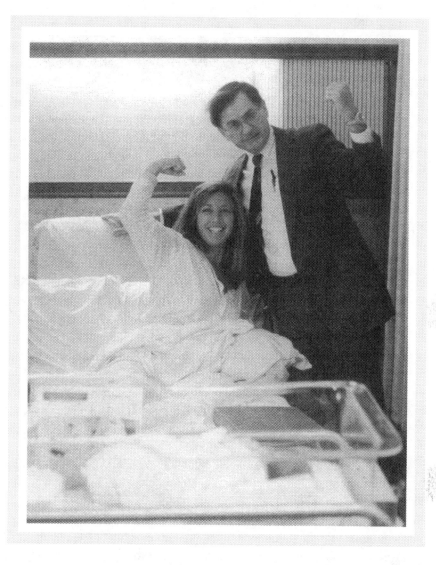

Here I am with my obstetrician, Dr. Giere, and, of course, Baby Kelly.

gradually build up over the next two to three weeks to a level that would be approximately the same as the level prior to your delivery.

Q. *What if you had a C-section?*

A. *With satisfactory recovery after a cesarean section, I would wait a little longer. If you would normally start with full activity after two to four weeks with a vaginal delivery, you may want to build up more slowly and be at full activity at four to six weeks. Remember, wait until you stop bleeding and have your doctor's approval.*

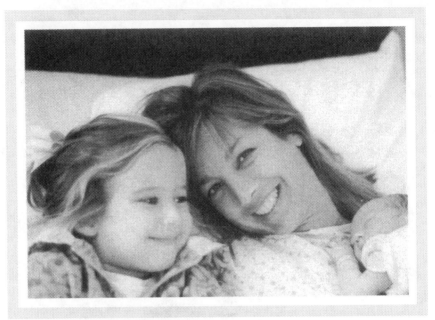

**Kelly's first sight of her new little sister,
just hours after she was born.**

Q. *When can you start doing aerobics again?*
A. *For an individual who has done aerobics before delivery, I think it is key to listen to your body. Begin slowly. You probably can begin two to four weeks after the delivery.*

Q. *What are the danger signals for a woman exercising postpartum?*
A. *Remember, the postpartum period is a very stressful time. Postpartum depression is not uncommon, and exercise is an excellent way to combat it. The new mother should watch her fatigue level, make sure that she gets whatever sleep she can obtain while caring for a newborn, watch the pattern of her bleeding, and also monitor other signs such as temperature or unusual pains—these would be the major things to watch out for.*

Q. *Technically, what happens to your abdominal muscles during pregnancy, and how do you get them back into shape?*
A. *The abdominal muscles are the muscles that extend from the breastbone to the pelvic bone, and during pregnancy they do stretch, become long and thin, and in certain cases they also may separate. After delivery, with*

exercise, they will return to their former shape, and the best exercise I can think of would be situps.

Q. *Is there any additional advice you would give new mothers?*
A. *I think I would tell them to pace themselves. Be realistic. Your body is a lot smarter than you think it is. Everyone says use common sense. Don't set too many tasks. Don't try to breast-feed quadruplets!*

FOR THE FIRST TWO WEEKS
AFTER THE BABY IS BORN

- **MINIMIZE YOUR SOCIAL VISITORS.**
- **HAVE SOMEONE ELSE DO ALL THE COOKING.**
- **TRUST YOUR INSTINCTS. MOTHERS SEEM TO KNOW. ALSO TRUST YOUR HUSBAND'S. GIVE HIM EVERY OPPORTUNITY TO FEED, BATHE, AND DIAPER THE BABY. JEFF ALWAYS DID GREAT, AND STILL DOES. BE A TEAM.**
- **DON'T THROW OUT THE MATERNITY CLOTHES YET.**
- **REALIZE THAT IT WILL TAKE THREE TO NINE MONTHS TO GET BACK INTO SHAPE.**

Immediately after your delivery, don't be shocked to look down and see a very gushy tummy. I'll never forget after I had my first baby, Kelly, I was in the hospital and I got up to go to the bathroom. For the first time I looked down at my abdomen. I just about died. It was so big and mushy! I looked about eight months pregnant.

No one ever warned me about that. I guess I honestly thought that after the baby came out, it would miraculously return to being flat. Boy, was I fooled. I had even bought cute outfits to go home in (one for me and one for the baby), and there was no way I could even dream of squeezing into mine.

One of my favorite memories was leaving the hospital with our new little sweetheart. I loved that event. I remember waking up that morning (not having slept more than two or three hours) and taking a shower for the first time. Nothing felt so good. It was the best shower of my life!

Jeff arrived, and we were both so excited. We got Kelly dressed and took a few pictures. They came with a wheelchair, and Jeff handed me Kelly. He wheeled us to the elevator, beaming with pride.

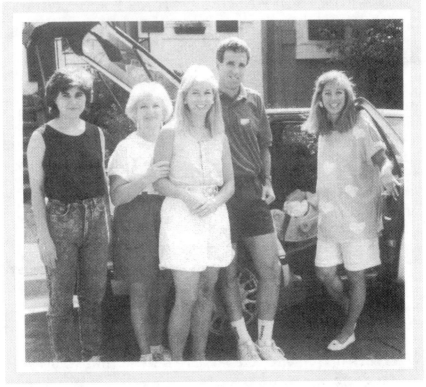

Home from the hospital!

As we left, a nun passed by and stopped to bless us (I delivered at Georgetown Hospital, which is Catholic), and I just started to cry. It was one of the most emotional and spiritual events of my life.

A FEW WORDS about nursing: "Breast is best."

By now you will have decided whether you will be breast-feeding your baby or bottle-feeding or a combination of both. I nursed my first child, Kelly, for nine months and my second daughter, Katie, for four months. (It just got harder with a three-year-old running around.) By the fourth week I also introduced both babies to one supplemental bot-

> My doctor recommended *sitz baths* (sitting on an inch or two of warm water) to relieve hemorrhoids and ease the pain of stitches, and they really helped.

tle a day, so Jeff could take over one nighttime feeding and I could get some rest.

Hopefully you will get a beautiful nightgown and robe to wear after the baby is born. My advice is to get one with buttons down the front so it's easier to whip out your breast to breast-feed. And blouses, too! It's so much easier when that baby is crying at the top of its lungs to be fed, and also less conspicuous.

If you are nursing, it is crucial for you to get all the nutrients your body needs. Don't skip meals. It will slow down your metabolism and drain your energy level.

Breast-feeding is not for everyone, so don't feel bad if you decide not to. Your baby will get all the nutrients he or she needs with formula.

Breast milk contains substances that protect the baby's immune system. Some of my best friends chose not to breast-feed, and they had wonderful, healthy children. As long as they are all nourished with tender love and care, babies will thrive whether breast- or bottle-fed. It's a very personal decision, and don't worry about the word "bonding" . . . you will have all the holding, rocking, and touching, stroking, and talking regardless of where the milk comes from. You will feel the bond in your own time. I did, and so did Jeff.

> *D*on't lose sleep over things you cannot change.
> Wash away guilt. Strive for a balance of health,
> fitness, nutrition, and happiness.

If you *do* decide to try breast-feeding, you will need to eat an additional **three hundred to five hundred calories a day.** That means three servings of protein, including chicken, fish, and other foods; two servings of foods high in vitamin C, five servings of calcium, three to six servings of fruits and veggies, six or more servings of complex carbohydrates, one or more serving of iron-rich foods like beef or beans, and your vitamin supplement for lactating women.

And you really can't drink enough **water** now. Every time I sat down to nurse, I had a giant glass of water beside me. It had to be finished when the baby was full.

Remember to put your feet up and put a pillow in your lap. (Jeff used to massage my neck, because it got sore from bending over to feed the baby.)

Or ask for one of those new Boppy Pillows as a shower gift.

Nursing burns **twenty calories** for every ounce you feed your baby. Some women can burn up to five hundred calories a day, but it is not a miracle cure for instantly getting back into shape.

Be patient!

And don't be alarmed if you experience a little cramping during nursing. It's a signal that your uterus is tightening up to its prepregnancy size (about the size of a pear). I personally felt that nursing helped me return to my prepregnancy shape more quickly. Unfortunately, studies show that breast-feeding can actually make you hold on to your body fat even though you look better and your uterus is shrinking. But don't worry—after you stop nursing you'll be amazed to drop four to ten pounds in one week. Remember, your baby is worth the wait!

Nursing is a great way to "jump start" your after-baby shape-up!

When my nipples got sore, I would break open a capsule of vitamin E and rub them gently. Lanolin also works great. Most important, I would let them air dry, (when no one was around!) by keeping my shirt open as long as possible after breast-feeding. I have also learned that many women find comfort in **cabbage leaves,** pressed to their breasts. Take two large leaves and microwave them for about fifteen seconds. Place one on each breast.

Nursing does get easier after the third week. Try sticking it out. Don't give up. It honestly becomes painless very quickly.

Also, here's a neat trick to help you remember which breast you last had the baby nurse from. I usually started on my right and then switched to my left. But sometimes the baby would fall asleep before finishing, so I took one pierced earring (it was a small pearl stud) and wore it on my right earlobe if I *last* nursed my right breast or my left one if I finished on my left side. You can't imagine how many times that saved me. (Yes, we are still a little absentminded now, with all the changes going on and the interrupted sleep!)

If you don't have pierced ears, switch your watch or bracelet. Another commonly used idea is putting a safety pin in the bra strap of the breast you nursed with last.

If you feel you need help with any breast-feeding questions, there are great resources. Call (800) LA LECHE or check out its Web site (http://www.laleche-league.org/). Also, purchase several breast-feeding books and use two or three books as resources. It is very comforting to read the same advice twice or to compare differing theories.

• • •

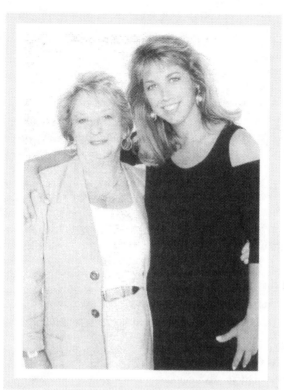

MY MOTHER (WHO lives three thousand miles away) and I talk on the phone almost every day. She means the world to me, and I can't imagine life without her. We're very lucky to enjoy such a close relationship. She has always been my biggest source of support and encouragement. Talk to your mother about how you were as a child. It's fun to hear these stories. Or maybe ask your mother-in-law about how your husband was as a child. . . . How much did he weigh at birth? It's fun to get out your and your husband's baby pictures and compare them with your newborn.

For those of you who have parents or in-laws that seem always to give unwanted advice, be patient. They just want to be involved. Gently remind them that it was more than twenty years ago since they had babies or young children. Memories fade.

I always wanted children, but not until I actually had my own did I realize that I could love a child so much. Every parent says this, and it's true. And when they start to form their own personalities and talk and then say, "I love you, Mommy," it's worth everything. I can't imagine going through life without having children and raising a family. It's the only thing that matters when it comes right down to it.

You are blessed now with your new baby. Your nurturing instincts will help you become a wonderful mother. And remember . . . motherhood is forever.

> *P*ay special attention to your husband now. He might be feeling a little jealous of all the attention you're paying the baby. Make him feel needed, loved, and appreciated. Resist the urge to take all the credit.

SEVEN TIPS TO ENHANCE YOUR BODY'S HEALING

1. Eat the right foods.
2. Stay active throughout the day.
3. Use relaxation techniques five minutes a day.
4. Drink plenty of water.
5. Focus on the spiritual aspects of life.
6. Spend time with people you love and who raise your spirits.
7. Visualize yourself in that "little black dress." See it to believe it!

Three weeks after the baby is born . . . Clean out your closet! Let's get rid of all those big maternity clothes, saving a few pairs of elastic-waist pants or skirts. You'll need a little extra breathing room while you get back into shape.

Four weeks after the baby is born . . . Schedule a hair appointment. Now's the time to get that color or permanent and a good trim. You need a little pampering after all that mothering. And don't forget to bring the baby pictures!

You may notice you've lost some hair since the baby was born. This usually occurs two to five months after birth and is nothing to worry about. As your hormones are changing, your hair might appear to be "shedding." This is only temporary; your hair will return to its normal growing pattern after some time. For some people, their hair never really fills in.

If you don't have the time or money for a facial, treat yourself to my **minifacial.** It's a great stress reliever, and we often overlook our faces when we think of massaging our bodies. Try to do this every day while the baby naps.

- **PLACE YOUR INDEX FINGERS AT THE INSIDE CORNERS OF YOUR EYES, ON EITHER SIDE OF THE BRIDGE OF YOUR NOSE.**
- **MAKE SMALL CIRCLES ON YOUR SKIN; KEEP MAKING SMALL CIRCLES AS YOU WORK YOUR INDEX FINGERS ALL THE WAY AROUND YOUR EYES.**
- **MAKE THREE SMALL CIRCLES OVER EACH TEMPLE. MAKE THREE CIRCLES FROM THE MIDDLE OF YOUR FOREHEAD OUT AND UP TOWARD YOUR HAIRLINE.**
- **REPEAT TWICE.**
- **MASSAGE YOUR CHEEKS AND JAWS WITH YOUR THUMBS AND THE PADS OF YOUR FINGERTIPS—GENTLY, GENTLY.**
- **RUB SMALL SECTIONS OF SKIN WITH LIGHT, QUICK MOTIONS, STARTING AT THE CHIN AND MOVING UP AND OUT ALONG THE CHEEKS AND JAW, FOR A COUNT OF TEN.**

This exercise not only releases tension, it improves your postpregnancy complexion by increasing circulation to your skin, and it feels fantastic! Also, I like to use my favorite moisturizer or scented body lotion for this minifacial. Close your eyes and picture yourself at a salon.

Dear Denise

What is a realistic amount of time to expect to get back into shape after the baby is born?

Three to nine months is about normal, in my experience, sooner rather than later if you followed through in eating right and exercising throughout your pregnancy. Right after you deliver, you should expect to lose about three to fifteen pounds. That makes up the weight of the baby, the placenta, the amniotic fluid, and blood loss.

You will still be carrying some material stores of fluids and fats. Your uterine muscles are still stretched, which is why you still look pregnant!

Don't worry. It will be taut again after you do your exercises, and time heals all.

I looked good after four months, but honestly, it took nine months to really get back into the greatest shape . . . we are all so critical of ourselves. I just thought of it as nine months of pregnancy and nine months back to a perfect fit!

So give yourself time!

•   •   •

OVER THE YEARS I've learned a few tricks to hide a thick waistline or "pouchy" tummy. You don't have to wear a size six to find flattering styles. And now that you are recovering from childbirth, there are plenty of ways to complement your figure. Colorful boxy jackets or double-breasted styles that fall just below your hips are a great choice now, especially when paired with elastic-waist soft skirts. Stay away from clingy knits. Sweaters that fall below the tummy and hips are also a good choice. And don't think you have to stick to basic black to look slim. Consider sapphire blue, emerald green, or ruby red as an alternative.

To instantly whittle your middle:

- **CHOOSE DRESSES WITH EMPIRE BODICES; THEY DRAW ATTENTION UP AND AWAY FROM THE WAIST.**
- **ANY V NECKLINE IS GOOD; THE DEEPER THE V, THE LONGER THE LINE.**
- **TRY TAILORED PANTS WITH A CLASSIC FIT. NARROW LEGS AND SIDE OR BACK ZIPPERS ARE ALSO A GOOD CHOICE. BAGGY PANTS NEVER FOOL ANYONE.**
- **CONSIDER A POLO SWEATER WITH A BANDED BOTTOM; IT WILL COVER TUMMY BULGES AND DRAW ATTENTION UPWARD.**
- **PUT ON A SHIRTDRESS AND CAMOUFLAGE A THICK MIDDLE.**
- **REMEMBER THAT A-LINE SKIRTS CREATE THE ILLUSION OF A NIPPED-IN MIDDLE.**
- **SHEATH DRESSES, WITH MATCHING JACKET OR HIP-LENGTH SWEATER, ARE EFFECTIVE. A SINGLE COLOR IS MOST SLIMMING. THE DRESS COVERS A THICK WAIST, AND THE JACKET OR SWEATER HIDES HIPS AND REAR END.**
- **WEAR A PAIR OF CONTROL-TOP PANTY HOSE!**

Instant slimmer . . . Try this trick I learned from a fashion stylist at a photo shoot. Tuck your top into your panty hose and smooth down before sliding on skirts on pants. It prevents the material from bunching up and adding bulk around your tummy, hips, and rear end.

WHAT TO STAY AWAY FROM

- **GATHERED SKIRTS: THE FABRIC WILL BULGE JUST WHERE YOU LEAST NEED IT TO, AT OR BELOW THE WAIST.**
- **JACKETS BELTED AT THE WAIST: TOO BULKY.**

- **SKIMPY, TIGHT TOPS.**
- **HORIZONTAL STRIPES AND DESIGNS.**
- **FLY FRONT CLOSINGS.**

Q. *Now that the baby is here, I seem to be fatigued and irritable. Is this normal?*

A. *Motherhood places enormous pressure on women, especially in this day and age when we are supposed to be "superwomen." Well, that is a myth. Your goal should be to have a happy, healthy family life, and that means setting priorities, planning, and balancing. Make a pact to create a positive environment within your home. You are the heart of the home. A smile goes a long way, and a cheerful atmosphere will affect everyone around you. Getting enough rest, eating right, and exercising will improve your mood. So will realizing that not everything will get done now that you have a baby to take care of. Let go of your old standards.*

Jeff and I waited seven years before starting our family. It was a wonderful time to establish our marriage first, before having children. Once I had my baby, things did change, and it's all worth it. Some days I wonder if the pace of motherhood keeps me from getting enough done or if life is passing me by.

But then Kelly will get on the phone while I'm away on a business trip and say, "I love you bigger than the whole sky," and I will tear up with joy.

So try to be patient now, as you learn to adjust your life to your baby's schedule. Be kind to yourself and not overly critical. And remember, don't take on more than you have the energy for. Scale back your commitments. Let the laundry pile up. Don't try to keep the kitchen spotless. Parenthood can be overwhelming at first. Some days I didn't even have time to get out of my pajamas.

Give yourself permission to fail sometimes. Try to simplify your life. The important things will get done. Here are five tricks I learned to keep my busy schedule in order:

1. *Use Sunday to plan for the week ahead.*
2. *Keep a calendar on the fridge.*
3. *Try to exercise in the morning, before the day's activities begin.*
4. *Ask for help if you need it. Learn to delegate.*
5. *Prepare meals in advance and freeze them.*

If you have a baby-sitter full- or part-time, ask her to run the errands for you, like getting the milk and diapers, picking up dry cleaning, and stopping at the pharmacy. Stay with your baby and have others do the chores.

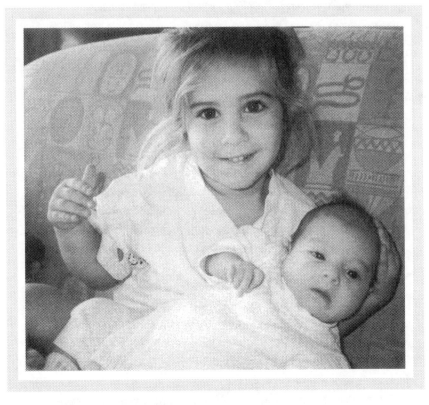

Big sister, little sister . . .

*If you don't have help, ask relatives and friends or maybe pool your re-
sources. After my second baby was born, I actually couldn't wait to go to the
grocery store (just to get out of the house!). So I asked a friend to come over,
and she watched the girls while I ran out. When I came back, she left to do her
errands and I watched her kids, and the older children had a blast together.*

*On a more serious note, postpartum depression is very real. We have all
gotten a little bit down because of the changing hormones, feeling tired, and
also feeling alone and isolated. It's normal. But if you think it's more
serious, call your doctor.*

Q. *I've seen advertisements for new miracle stretch mark creams. Do they
really work?*

A. *Stretch marks appear when the skin's deeper layers—collagen and elastin—
are stretched by weight gain, and they break down. Pregnant women are
likely to get them. Any moisturizer can make your skin more supple looking,
but the effect is usually temporary. At the moment, no "miracle" cream on
the market has been scientifically proved to erase or fade stretch marks. One*

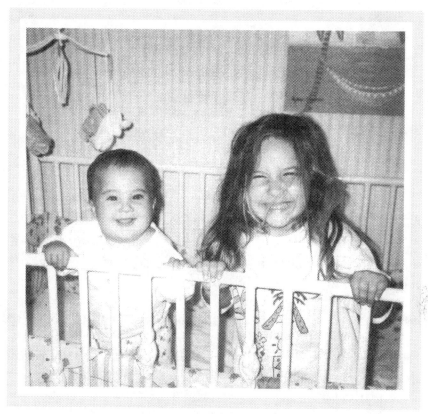

My precious girls . . .

recent study showed that Retin-A, in concentrated prescription form, did help fade new pink and purplish stretch marks. It also caused stinging and redness. Ask your doctor to recommend a cream if your stretch marks are unusually swollen or purple. Be careful if you are nursing. What you put on your skin is absorbed into the body. And as always, be patient! They will likely fade in the next six months, as your body returns to its normal shape.

Q. *I keep waking up in the middle of the night, drenched in perspiration. Is this normal?*

A. *Yes. I remember after my two babies were born, I sometimes woke up feeling totally damp with "night sweats." In the weeks following delivery, your body will begin to lose water it had been retaining during your last trimester, and this is nothing to be alarmed about. It also means you are starting to lose more of the pregnancy weight. I slept in all-cotton nightshirts, and sometimes I put a towel under me, just in case. But it's important to keep hydrated, so don't be afraid to keep drinking your water!*

CHAPTER 11

Lose That "Baby Fat"

*D*on't be surprised if you are as hungry now as you were during the second trimester of your pregnancy. Suddenly food tastes wonderful (oh, those hormones), and if you are nursing, your dietery needs are just as important as before the baby was born.

It's important for lactating mothers to understand that flavors of the foods they eat can cross over into breast milk. Sometimes we learn it the hard way. I remember nursing Kelly one morning after eating broccoli the night before. I didn't realize that it would make her fussy, which it did. She cried for a while, and a friend told me it was probably the broccoli, which, like onions, is gassy. I never even thought of that.

Katie was different. I could eat anything, and she was fine. But Kelly was definitely more colicky, especially from five to eight P.M. I tried to eat bland foods and drink plenty of water.

It won't take long for you to figure out which foods are too strong for your baby to handle. And remember, if you decide to breast-feed, save the champagne for later. It's crucial for nursing mothers to continue to avoid alcohol and caffeine. You're not on your own again yet!

If you are not nursing, you can begin to lower your calorie intake gradually. Crash diets are not the answer. You need your strength to take care of your infant, and skipping meals will only make you weak and irritable. Eat sensibly. Choose a balanced diet of protein, complex carbohydrates, fruits, and veggies, and continue to drink your milk!

Remember:

- **DON'T SKIP BREAKFAST.**
- **NO CRASH DIETS.**
- **BOOST YOUR VITAMIN B INTAKE.**
- **EAT FIVE A DAY—FRUITS AND VEGGIES.**

- **EIGHT GLASSES OF WATER.**
- **WALK FOR THIRTY MINUTES.**

Only a combination of diet and exercise can take off pounds, and we want to do this slowly and steadily. Remember, you are forming lifelong eating habits, which will help you maintain your ideal weight, have more energy, and look and feel your best.

AFTER-BABY ENERGY-BOOSTING STRATEGY

For breakfast, try to eat whole-grain cereals with skim milk, fruit, and a glass of orange juice. For your snack, stick to nonfat yogurt and fruit. For lunch, nothing is better than a sliced turkey sandwich with lettuce, tomato, and mustard, along with a cup of vegetable or lentil soup. For dinner, plan on skinless, boneless chicken breasts, fresh vegetables and a salad (low-fat dressing), and a sweet potato or baked potato.

Did you know . . . that two French fries from a fast-food restaurant are equal in fat to two whole baked potatoes ($\frac{1}{2}$ gram fat)? One corn chip is equal to forty baby carrots (1 gram fat)? One ounce of potato chips is equal to twenty ounces of pretzels (10 grams fat)?

Many people ask me exactly what I eat to stay fit. Believe me, I'm not perfect. But I try to eat healthfully 80 percent of the time, and the other 20 percent of the time I allow myself to indulge in treats. If you overeat on special occasions such as holidays, enjoy it! Food is fabulous. The key

Instead of	Choose . . .
White bread	Bread labeled 100 percent stone-ground whole-wheat
White flour crackers	Crackers with 20 grams of fiber per serving
White rice	Brown rice or quinoa
Sugary cereals	Cereals with at least 5 grams of fiber per serving: oatmeal, Raisin Bran, Shredded Wheat

is not to punish yourself for the infrequent slipups, because then you'll fall into a negative cycle. Wake up the next day with a fresh slate. Eat wisely, and you will eat well.

After I stopped nursing, I stuck to a 1,500-calorie diet, consuming about 20 percent fat. Eating smart is the answer—not denying yourself!

I keep cut up raw veggies in the refrigerator to avoid heavy snacking and try to eat dinner by eight P.M. every night. Eat dinner as early as possible.

I also stay away from refined carbohydrates such as white bread. The fiber is removed in the milling process. Unrefined carbohydrates, such as whole-grain foods, keep their fiber.

You need a wide variety of foods in your life. Look at your eating habits on a weekly basis. Vary your diet for more satisfying meals.

Here is a sample of what I might eat during a typical day:

Breakfast (300 calories)

⅔ cup Muesli

8 ounces skim milk

Small banana

Lunch (511 calories)

2 ounces sliced turkey breast with 1-ounce low-fat

Swiss cheese and romaine lettuce, tomato, sprouts,

and Dijon mustard on 2 slices pumpernickel bread

Glass of skim milk

Fresh navel orange

Snack (60 calories)

1 fruit choice (apple, 1 cup cantaloupe, ½ grapefruit,

15 grapes, 2 tablespoons raisins)

Dinner (500 calories)

*½ cup Progresso White Clam Sauce over 3 ounces fresh
  linguine*

*1 large broccoli spear, steamed with a squeeze of fresh
  lemon*

12 fresh cherries

Dessert (100 calories)

1 sliver angel food cake

After I stopped nursing, I did treat myself to an occasional margarita or glass of white wine.

Did you know . . . that ounce for ounce, **hard cheeses** contain almost as much protein as lean beef? Although it is higher in calories and fat than beef, cheese is a wonderful flavor booster. I confess, I love crumbled blue cheese on salads, and warm mozzarella drizzled with olive oil on a slice of Italian bruschetta. I like to sprinkle grated Parmesan on microwave popcorn for a low-calorie, rich-tasting snack. But I have to be careful, sometimes, not to overdo it.

> **Nursing mothers need to take in a minimum of 1,000 milligrams of calcium each day. The best way is through dairy products, low-fat or reduced-fat cheese, and leafy greens.**

The good news is that reduced-fat cheese exists—and some even have more calcium than full-fat cheeses.

Even among full-fat cheeses, you'd be surprised to know that creamy rich Brie cheese is slightly lower in fat than cheddar cheese. Here's a chart that shows that ounce for ounce, no two cheeses are alike.

Calcium-rich Cheeses

One Ounce

Parmesan	335 milligrams
Romano	300 milligrams
Gruyère	290 milligrams
Swiss	270 milligrams
Provolone	210 milligrams
Mozzarella, part skim	205 milligrams
Cheddar	205 milligrams

Grams of Fat per Ounce

Cheddar	9 grams
Monterey jack	9 grams
American	9 grams
Swiss	8 grams
Provolone	8 grams
Jarlsberg	7.0 grams
Camembert	7.0 grams
Neufchâtel	6.5 grams
Feta	6.0 grams
Goat cheese	6.0 grams
Mozzarella, part skim	5.5 grams

While I was nursing, I used to love different grilled cheese sandwiches for lunch (low-fat sharp cheddar and tomato, melted with a little chutney) or spreading ricotta cheese on a slice of nut bread for an afternoon snack. Cheese is a great source of calcium, protein, and vitamin A.

A word about low-fat cheeses: Watch the sodium content! One slice of low-fat single American processed cheese can contain up to 466 milligrams of sodium, so read the labels carefully before buying.

Six weeks after the baby is born... Now's the time when many of us have to return to work. More than half of all new mothers return to the workforce, and I know how hard it can be. I had to be ready to film my television show six weeks after each of my daughters was born. (At least *you* don't have to get back into a leotard!) But I was also fortunate to have the opportunities to travel with my two babies. I look back and think, How did I do it? It can be a traumatic time, trying to juggle all the responsibilities. But so many of us do it. You can, too.

I reserved Sunday afternoon for planning time. That's when Jeff and I would sit down and go over our calendar, planning the week. I also learned to plan the week's meals by shopping for the right foods, then precooking and freezing certain dishes. It really helped. Not everything can be frozen, and sometimes we do have the time to prepare dinner. But I liked to have a few things on hand to avoid panic in the early evening, especially if Jeff was out for a business dinner and Kelly was colicky.

Here's a sample meal plan for nursing moms.

Breakfast

A breakfast sandwich:

Scrambled egg with a slice of provolone cheese on an
English muffin

A cup of hot cocoa (with skim milk)

½ grapefruit

Midmorning

1 cinnamon graham rectangle

Juice sparkler: 4 ounces white grape juice with 8 ounces
seltzer water

Lunch

A tuna pita:

3 ounces water-packed tuna mixed with 1 tablespoon
*   light mayonnaise*

Lettuce and tomato

1 whole-grain 6-inch pita

8 ounces lemon water

1 pear

Midafternoon

1 granola bar

8 ounces skim milk

Dinner

2 cups beef stew made with lean beef, vegetables,
*   potatoes, and beef bouillon*

A salad with 2 tablespoons light vinaigrette

1 small roll with 1 teaspoon whipped butter

8 ounces water

Total

Calories: 2,109

Fat: 60 grams

Carbohydrates 55 percent, Protein 20 percent, Fat
*   25 percent*

Here's a sample meal plan for nonnursing moms to lose weight.

Breakfast

¾ cup cereal (flake type or toasted oats) with
   ¼ cup crunchy cereal on top
6 ounces skim milk
5-inch banana

Midmorning

1 rice cake with 1 tablespoon peanut butter

Lunch

Club sandwich on a bagel:
Slice a bagel into three parts:
on ⅓ put a slice of turkey breast or 2 thin deli slices
on ⅓ put a slice of bacon and lettuce
on ⅓ put 1 slice of tomato and 1 tablespoon light
   mayonnaise
1 orange cut into wedges

Midafternoon

3 cups microwave light popcorn or 3 cups air-popped
   popcorn with 1 tablespoon Parmesan cheese
8 ounces seltzer water

Dinner

Stuffed shells:

Sauté 1 package frozen spinach in 2 teaspoons olive oil.

Mix in a 12-ounce container of low-fat ricotta cheese.

*Spoon 2 tablespoons of spinach mixture into cooked
    jumbo shells (yields ten to twelve).*

*Pour spaghetti sauce over shells and bake at
    350 degrees for 25 minutes.*

Serving size: 2 shells.

with

*Crudités: baby carrots, sliced cucumbers, and
    pepper strips (about 1½ cups)*

*1 cup fresh or frozen unsweetened berries with 2
    tablespoons nondairy light topping*

Total

Calories: 1,598

Fat: 44 grams

*Carbohydrates 55 percent, Protein 21 percent,
    Fat 24 percent*

Here are a few recipes I enjoyed in the months after my babies were born. They are high in protein and minerals and low in calories. They are easy to prepare, and some can be made ahead of time and either refrigerated or frozen.

Warm Chicken Salad with Oranges

(Serves 4)

■

The oranges give this salad a light, citrusy flavor and an added calcium and vitamin C boost! This is also one of the quickest meals in my recipe file.

½ POUND FRESH SNOW PEAS

2 BONELESS CHICKEN BREASTS

FLOUR TO COAT

1 TABLESPOON VEGETABLE OIL

SALAD GREENS

2 FRESH SEEDLESS FLORIDA ORANGES, PEELED AND SECTIONED

¼ CUP SLICED SCALLIONS

1 TABLESPOON LIME JUICE

1 TABLESPOON ORANGE JUICE

½ CUP SEEDLESS GREEN GRAPES, HALVED

2 TEASPOONS DIJON MUSTARD

1 TABLESPOON OLIVE OIL

In a pot of boiling water, place snow peas. Blanch for two minutes, then plunge peas into bowl of ice water to stop the cooking process. Drain and set aside.

Pound chicken breasts on cutting board with the back of your hand, and coat lightly with flour. Heat vegetable oil in skillet and add chicken, cooking about four minutes per side until nicely browned.

Arrange salad greens on plates. Slice the chicken breasts into thin strips and place on greens. Add snow peas, and arrange nicely.

To the warm skillet, add orange sections, scallions, lime juice, orange juice, grapes, and mustard. Simmer over low heat for several minutes. Stir in olive oil and blend over low heat for a few seconds with a spoon. Ladle orange sauce over chicken and snow peas.

Linguine with Asparagus and Shrimp

(Serves 4)

■

**This is a delicious main course, which supplies
5 milligrams of iron—one-third of your daily
requirement. And it takes almost no time to cook!**

2 TABLESPOONS OLIVE OIL
½ POUND FRESH SHRIMP, PEELED AND DEVEINED
½ POUND FRESH ASPARAGUS, BLANCHED AND DRAINED
JUICE OF 1 LEMON
1 POUND FRESH SPINACH LINGUINE
SALT AND PEPPER TO TASTE

Heat a large pot of salted water until boiling. While you wait, heat a few tablespoons olive oil in a large skillet over low to medium heat. Add shrimp and sauté for a few minutes, until the shrimp turns pink. Add the asparagus and lemon juice and toss lightly.

Boil the pasta according to package directions, drain, and transfer to the skillet. Toss with the shrimp and asparagus. Season with salt and pepper to taste. This can be served warm or made early in the day and served at room temperature.

Katie's Casserole

(Serves 4)

■

After my second daughter was born, I found I really looked for dishes I could freeze. This is one of our favorite ones, and the kids love it.

½ ONION, CHOPPED FINE
1 28-OUNCE CAN CHOPPED TOMATOES, WITH JUICE
1 1¼-OUNCE PACKAGE TACO MIX
1 15–16-OUNCE CAN BLACK BEANS, RINSED AND DRAINED
3 CUPS COOKED ZITI OR PENNE PASTA
(ABOUT 6 OUNCES DRIED)
1 CUP NONFAT RICOTTA CHEESE
½ POUND VERY LEAN GROUND BEEF, CRUMBLED
½ CUP NONFAT SHREDDED CHEDDAR CHEESE

Preheat oven to 425 degrees.

Spray a 7-by-11-inch baking dish with cooking spray. In a medium bowl or food processor, blend onion, tomatoes, taco mix, and black beans.

Spread 1 cup of the tomato sauce on the bottom of the baking dish. Add the cooked pasta. Dot with the ricotta and then spread cheese with a knife.

Stir the ground beef pieces into the remaining tomato sauce and spoon over the ricotta. Sprinkle with the shredded cheddar cheese. Bake twenty-five to thirty minutes.

Serve immediately or freeze. To reheat, bake at 350 degrees until top is bubbly, about thirty minutes.

Frozen Mousse Pie

(Serves 8)

∎

**None of my friends can believe that a dessert that
tastes this good can be low in fat and calories
(only 220 calories per serving and 5.5 grams of
fat). I used to make this on Sundays, freeze it, and
serve it all week, along with an extra one saved
for a dinner party. Your guests will love it.**

4 OUNCES BAKER'S SWEET CHOCOLATE
½ CUP SKIM MILK
8-OUNCE PACKAGE LIGHT CREAM CHEESE, SOFTENED
2 TABLESPOONS SUGAR
8-OUNCE CONTAINER LIGHT COOL WHIP
8-INCH OREO COOKIE CRUST

In a small saucepan, melt chocolate over very low heat with 2 table-spoons skim milk, stirring.

In a medium bowl, beat cream cheese with the sugar. Add remaining milk and blend in chocolate well. Gradually add light Cool Whip until all ingredients are incorporated. Spoon into cookie crust and freeze four to five hours before serving.

Congratulations! Because you need to keep well fueled and energized to nurse your little one, your calorie needs actually increase above needs during pregnancy. Aim for about 2,000 calories per day, as six easy-to-grab meals, and remember to keep up your fluid intake. Rest when you can, and eat well!

If you have decided to bottle-feed your baby, you can afford to cut back slightly on calories. The goal is *not* active weight loss, but a gradual steady loss to get back your prepregnancy shape. Remember, that little one requires a lot of energy, so you need to fuel well to meet the demands of motherhood! The calories can be around 1,600 per day, although I tried to stay at 1,500 a day.

CHAPTER 12

After-Baby Shape-up

*O*kay, we're ready to get back into shape!

Regardless of the joy that children bring, all mothers—no matter their age— are tired and physically worn out. That's why exercise is so important in the weeks and months following delivery. But just when you need to exercise the most, you find your time is limited. That's why it's so important now for you to decide to make the effort.

> *Y*ou don't know your capacity for love until
> you have a child.

One of the biggest tips I can give you now is to start back slowly into your exercise routine. I began doing **isometric exercises** right in the hospital, tightening and contracting the muscles, then relaxing.

Start with your tummy.

Pull in your belly button, tighten and contract your abdominal muscles for a count of three; then relax. Do about ten of these each day after a vaginal delivery.

Tighten your buttock muscles for three seconds, and release. Try to do ten of these each day.

Do a similar number of kegels each hour.

Pull in your abs and tilt your pelvis up and forward while straightening your back.

To improve your circulation, get moving and walk slowly for a few minutes three times a day. Straighten your spine and think of great posture.

You can do it!

To shed that weight and trim down fast, you need to attack the fat in three ways:

1. Eat a low-fat diet.
2. Burn fat through exercise, at least three times a week.
3. Tone and firm muscle at least twice a week to speed up your metabolism and to shape your abs, trim your waist, firm up your tush, and slim your hips and thighs.

I have divided this after-baby shape-up into three areas of fitness: aerobics (the walking program), toning (specific exercises to zero in on the tummy), plus a workout with weights and stretching for flexibility.

It takes only twenty to thirty minutes a day to make a real difference in your life and have the kind of healthy mind and body you deserve. This doesn't mean spending hours in the health club or gym or buying expensive machines. Personally, I walk for thirty to forty-five minutes Mondays, Wednesdays, and Fridays or do some form of aerobic exercise to burn the fat three days a week. Twice a week, Tuesdays and Thursdays, I do my thirty-minute toning routine to sculpt and firm the muscles and to fight the aging process.

I always leave a few minutes for stretching after my workouts. Stretching is relaxing, prevents soreness, and eases tension.

You can work out on your own, keeping your own schedule and following a simple plan of aerobic activity, stretches, and floor exercises.

Once you start, you will see the results almost immediately, and I will show you how to bounce back better than ever. Only thirty minutes a day . . . that's not so much to ask of yourself!

If you've had a normal, vaginal delivery and are feeling good, you can begin gentle exercises as soon as three days after childbirth. But remember, start slowly, talk to your doctor, and increase your activity gradually.

It would be nice to feel as though you can pick up right where you left off before the baby, but remember, you're going to have to walk before you run. Start gradually.

Now is also the time to check out my *Bounce Back After Baby* video. It's a best-seller, and there's reason for that: It really works. Every week I get letters from women telling me how easy and fun it was and how grateful they are.

> Exercise is my mental filter; it filters out all my anxieties and makes me feel relaxed and energized . . . and fun to be around!

KEGELS	**10-second hold**
TUMMY TUCKS	**Breathing in, then tightening.** **Pull in tummy. Release and repeat.** **Lie on your back, slight pelvic tilt.**
POSTURE PERFECT	**Bring your shoulder blades back** **together while doing a pelvic tilt.** **Do standing, back against the wall.**
SHOULDER ROLL	**Roll the shoulders forward 5 times** **and back 5 times.**

I get excited when I read success stories. But don't judge yourself by anyone else's progress. It took me about three to four months to lose my thirty-five pounds, but it may take you longer to lose your weight, and you may have moments of feeling discouraged, when you think you can't do it. But you can!

The biggest obstacle to exercising is time. You must decide today to make time whenever you can.

Raising a family certainly puts demands on your time, so learn to squeeze in exercise any time you can. The next time you talk on the phone, use your other arm to firm up the **triceps.** How? Lift one arm overhead. Slowly bend your elbow and then straighten it out again. Keep your arm close to your ear.

Do **standing leg lifts** while washing dishes or standing in front of the stove or at the changing table.

My philosophy has always been to turn idle time into toning time. Plus, you get great results in firming, doing a minute here and a minute there. That's the beauty of toning. Your muscles don't know if you're in a gym or your kitchen.

Aerobic exercise is different. For best results, aerobics need to be done in a chunk of time, preferably at least twenty to thirty minutes straight, to get your heart rate up and burn fat.

Walking is a great way to get back into shape. Try my postpartum walking workout, described later in this chapter.

If you miss a few days of exercise, don't beat yourself up. Just do your best to be active anyway and then get back on track and plan to fit a good workout into the next day. Schedule it. Put in on your calendar. Make an

> My workout conforms with the guidelines set by the American College of Obstetricians and Gynecologists. But consult your OB/GYN before starting any exercise program.

appointment with yourself or with a friend, and give yourself the gift of fitness.

Tip: Get out of your pajamas as quickly as you can so you don't feel lazy.

Now you're ready for my after-baby workout!

So pick out a bright leotard, put on your sneakers, and let's go!

- **PERFORM EXERCISES ON A WOODEN FLOOR OR TIGHTLY CARPETED SURFACE TO PREVENT SLIPPING.**
- **NEVER OVERSTRETCH. JOINTS ARE STILL EXTREMELY FLEXIBLE.**
- **TAKE LIQUIDS BEFORE, DURING, AND AFTER EXERCISE TO PREVENT DEHYDRATION.**
- **TAKE YOUR TIME. THE PHYSIOLOGICAL CHANGES OF PREGNANCY REMAIN IN YOUR SYSTEM SIX TO TWELVE MONTHS POSTPARTUM. HORMONES WILL NOT RETURN TO NORMAL UNTIL BREAST-FEEDING IS STOPPED.**

IF YOU ARE BREAST-FEEDING

Always breast-feed your baby first and then exercise. This is for two reasons:

1. You will be more comfortable exercising if your breasts are not full.
2. Sometimes if you breast-feed immediately after exercising, the baby can be fussy. Some studies have shown that babies sometimes reject the lactic acid taste of postexercise breast milk. However, my babies *never* did.

Be sure to wear a good, supportive bra that fits snugly. Don't be afraid to wear two bras if you need to. However, take your bra(s) off immediately after exercise. Keep your breasts as clean and dry as possible. You don't want your milk ducts to become clogged, which can cause an infection.

For my aerobic activity after the birth of my babies, I started with twenty-minute walks while I was strolling them. I gradually increased my pace and duration until I got up to forty-five minutes three times a week. On some days I walked alone or with a friend and picked up the pace even more, to a brisk trot. I also used my own video to do aerobic exercises at home. Sometimes I'd just put on fun music and dance, holding my baby against me in the Snugli!

I also used to get a workout, right in the privacy of my home, by putting the baby in the baby swing and doing my aerobics in front of her. I remember she would stare at me while I did the quick thirty-minute routine, and she loved the music and the movements.

HERE IS A six-week postpartum walking workout to shed your baby fat!

Begin only with medical clearance from your doctor. If at any time during your walk you feel exhausted or uncomfortable, stop and rest.

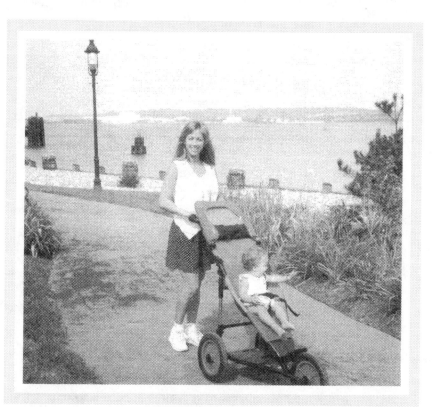

Walking with your child is great. Here I am with Katie.

By embarking on a regular walking plan—like the one outlined here—you can gradually walk your way back to your prepregnancy weight. I promise!

TIPS FOR POSTPARTUM WALKERS

1. Buy a good pair of walking shoes that fits properly, especially since your feet have changed size.
2. Walk first thing in the morning, before breakfast, if incontinence is still a problem. In freezing weather or in the evening, a treadmill might be a better option.
3. Take a water bottle with you, especially if you are nursing. Feed the baby before you walk.
4. Use headphones only if you are not with the baby. Since you're a mom now, be extra careful crossing streets, and keep the volume low enough so that you can still hear what's going on around you.
5. Pump your arms (keeping them at chest level) to help increase your heart rate and burn more calories.

Many new mothers find it's easy to take the baby along. I love my baby jogger. I always get a bunch of girls together and pitch in to buy one for baby showers . . . it's the best present!

If you decide to walk while strolling the baby—which will burn more calories than simply walking alone—remember a few safety tips:

1. Don't wear headphones. It's important not to be distracted while walking/strolling.
2. Always set the rear wheel parking brake if you are not in control of the stroller.
3. Dress the baby a little more warmly than you. The baby is not exercising. You are!
4. Bring along water for yourself, and diapers, juice, and wipes for the baby, and a portable telephone never hurts!

POSTPARTUM WALKING WORKOUT

Begin your workout only after you've gotten medical clearance from your doctor. If at any time during your walk you feel exhausted or uncomfortable, slow down and rest. You may customize this workout according to your own fitness level by increasing or decreasing the frequency, speed, time, or distance.

- **REMEMBER ALWAYS TO WARM UP SLOWLY AND COOL DOWN AFTER YOUR WALK BY STROLLING FOR SEVERAL MINUTES.**

Week	Days/Wk.	MPH	Minutes	Miles	Goals
1	3–5	3.0	10	0.5	Get used to light exercise, and begin to regain a sense of control of your body. Speed, time, and distance are not important.
2	3–5	3.0	15	0.8	Establish a regular time. Keep a steady pace.
3	4–5	3.0	20	1.0	A 20-minute mile and increased frequency. If you are feeling sore or your joints are hurting, take a day off. Try adjusting the length of your stride or reducing speed if you feel pelvic, joint, or mammary pain. (See a doctor if pain is persistent.)

(continued)

Week	Days/Wk.	MPH	Minutes	Miles	Goals (cont.)
4	5	3.5	25	1.4	Increase speed, distance, and time for a higher calorie burn.
5	5	3.5	30	1.7	Pass the "talk test." You should be breathing hard but still be able to carry on a conversation.
6	5	4.0	30	2.0	A 15-minute mile. Continue to improve fitness level by increasing intensity and/or duration. Your muscle tone will also improve, which helps burn more calories.

- **KEEP YOUR HEAD UP, SHOULDERS DOWN AND BACK, ABS PULLED IN, BUTT TUCKED IN.**
- **KEEP THE LENGTH OF YOUR STRIDE NATURAL, NOT JERKY OR FORCED.**
- **STOP IF THERE IS ANY PAIN.**

After week six continue walking five days per week. Burn more calories by increasing your speed, time, or mileage.

AFTER-BABY WORKOUT

These pictures were taken eight months after I gave birth to Katie, so don't feel bad. It might take you that long to bounce back better than before. You can do it! With effort, patience, and determination you can look and feel even better than you did before your pregnancy.

Tell yourself every day: You're worth it!

BOUNCE BACK WARM-UP

Put on your favorite music and begin to march in place. Pump your arms and legs for 3–5 minutes. Get moving!

If you have a treadmill or stationary bike, start to warm up your muscles and get your circulation going.

Don't you already feel *great?*

Bounce Back Tummy Flattener

Lie on your back (using an exercise mat for comfort, if you have one), bend your knees, and keep your feet flat on the floor. Flatten the small of your back against the floor, tilting your pelvis. Contract your abdominal muscles, exhale, and hold the position for 3–5 seconds. Relax and repeat.

REPEAT 2 sets of 8–12 reps.

BENEFITS: Works your abdominal muscles, builds a strong base of support for your back.

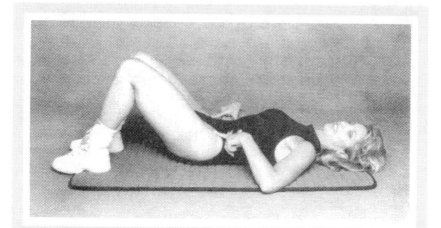

Bounce Back Tummy Tightener

Lie on your back, thighs perpendicular to your body, knees together, and legs extended, resting on a chair for support. Keep your feet straight. Legs should be at a 90-degree angle. Place your hands behind your head for support, tighten your abdominals, and simultaneously lift your head and shoulders about 6 inches from off the floor. Exhale. Can you feel the abdominals working? Slowly lower your shoulders back to the floor and repeat.

REPEAT 2 sets of 8–12 reps. Rest 15 seconds between sets.

BENEFITS: Lower and upper end of abdominals (rectus abdominis).

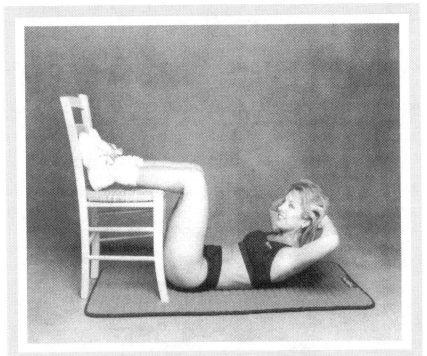

Bounce Back Lower Ab Tightener

Place a towel between your knees. Lift your hips up so pelvis is tilted and buttocks are off the floor a few inches. Relax and repeat.

REPEAT 2 sets of 8–12 reps.

BENEFITS: Trims and tightens the lower tummy and the inner thighs.

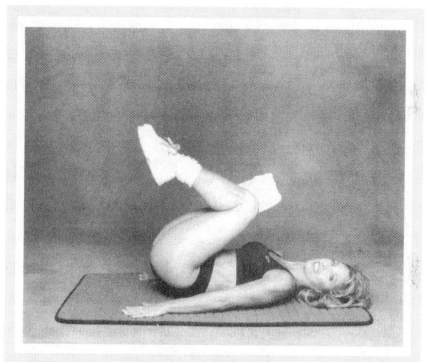

Bounce Back
Below-the-belly-button Firmer

Place a towel between your knees and feel more lower abs and inner thighs working. This exercise "zeros in" on the muscles closest to the pelvic bone and trims that after-baby pouchy tummy. Challenge yourself by keeping your legs straight. Contract the abdominal muscles, lifting your head and shoulders, and relax.

These are great exercises also for women who have had C-sections.

REPEAT 2 sets of 8–12 reps.

BENEFITS: Quickest way to bounce back is to strengthen those abs!

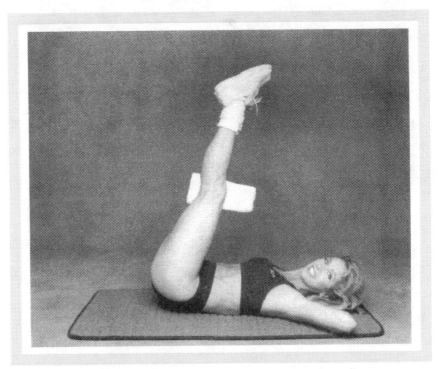

Bounce Back Total Ab Strengthener

.

This exercise involves most of the abdominal region. Think belly button in, lower back pressed to the floor, flat, hollow stomach. Lie on the floor with your right leg bent and your left leg bent and up. Keep your arms by your sides. Exhale as you pull your left knee toward your chest. Alternate legs. Continue to bicycle side to side, doing "toe taps" to the floor. Keep the movement smooth and flowing. Be sure to keep the lower back pressed into the floor and pull your abdomen in toward your spine.

REPEAT 2 sets of 8–12 reps. Rest 15 seconds between sets.

BENEFITS: Abdominals.

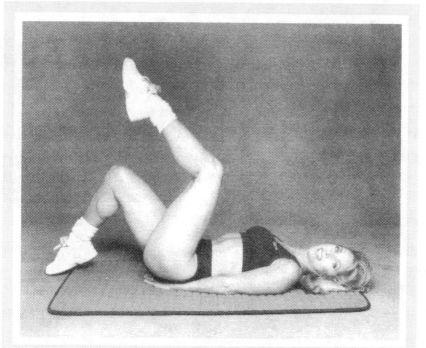

Bounce Back Waistline Whittle

This tummy-tightening crunch focuses on the internal and external obliques on the side of your tummy that support you laterally. As with all of our ab exercises, be sure that you try to contract your muscles with every rep. These will really help you get rid of those after-baby love handles!

Lie on the floor, bend your knees, and bring your left knee to your elbow. Bend and pull the knee toward the elbow and feel the "crunch." Switch sides and repeat.

REPEAT 2 sets of 8–12 reps.

BENEFITS: Trims the waist, tones and firms abdominals.

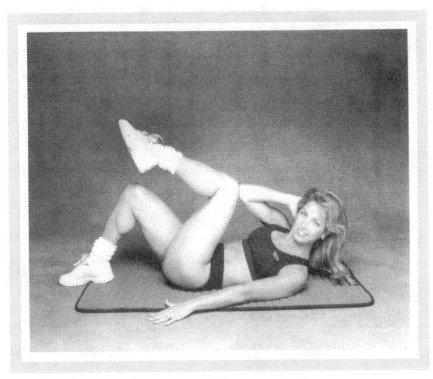

Bounce Back Lower Back Stretch

This exercise increases back flexibility, reduces pressure on your back (especially from fatigue and after-baby emotional tension), and cools you down.

Lie on your back, bend your knees to your chest, and bear hug, grasping hands under thighs. Press the small of the back against the floor, keep your abdomen flat, and pretend that the naval is pressing into your spine. Hold for 15–20 seconds, breathing deeply, and relax.

REPEAT 2 sets of 8–12 reps.

BENEFITS: Relaxes the muscles, eases tension.

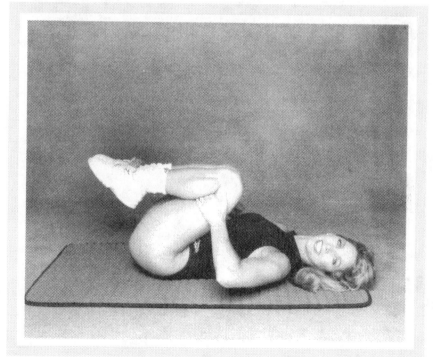

Bounce Back Spine Strengthener

Lie on the floor, with your elbows bent. Stretch your legs out straight, toes pointed. Feel your abdominal muscles elongate and stretch. This is also a great tension reliever. This is a great exercise to do after your ab work.

REPEAT 2 sets of 8–12 reps.

BENEFITS: The spine, increases flexibility. Posture improver!

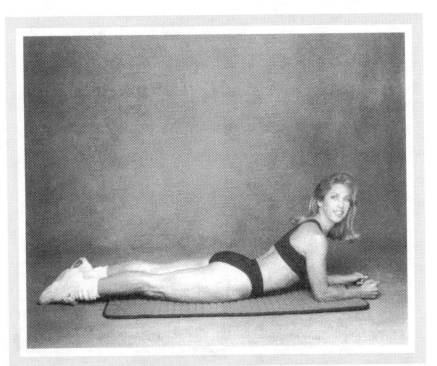

Bounce Back Bottoms Up

This is a great exercise for the legs and one of my favorites. Stand up straight, arms outstretched. Now slowly lower your bottom to a chair. Feel as though you are sitting back, with your body's weight in your heels. Do this one in front of a mirror, using the chair, until you get the hang of it. Watch your form!

REPEAT 2 sets of 8–12 reps.

BENEFITS: Works three different muscle groups: the quadriceps (front of the leg), the hamstrings (back of the leg), and the gluteals (the muscles in your buttocks).

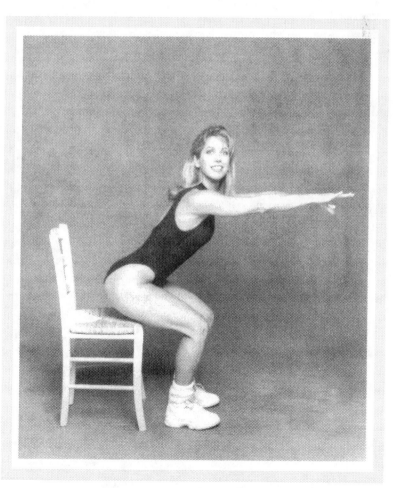

Bounce Back Lower Body Total Toner

·

This is one of the most effective exercises you can do to work the *entire* leg. Lunges can be done with no weights at all, whole holding dumbells or with a bar on your shoulders. If you do add weights, increase their size gradually.

Start with one foot in front of the other, using a chair for balance. Lower yourself, bending both knees, making sure your knee stays in line with your ankle. Your weight should be on your back toes and on your front heel. Straighten legs until you are standing, and lower yourself again. Watch your form! Don't let your front knee extend over the front of your toes. Repeat with opposite leg.

REPEAT 16–24 reps.

BENEFITS: Tones and strengthens your lower body.

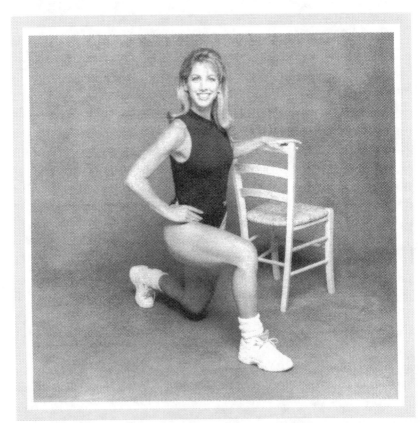

Bounce Back Hip and Thigh Slimmer

This is a terrific exercise for your outer thighs. As you do this exercise, make sure you don't swing your leg—move deliberately and concentrate on the outer part of your thigh.

Stand with one hand on a chair for balance. Slowly raise your leg and lower it to the floor. This is a short movement, and you should feel the resistance in your outer thigh. Repeat, and switch legs.

REPEAT 2 sets of 8–12 reps for each leg.

BENEFITS: No more saddlebags!

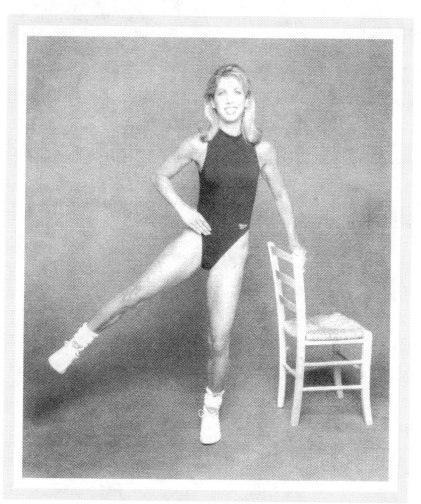

Bounce Back Inner Thigh Trimmer

This is the same idea as the previous exercise. Stand, using a chair for balance. Move one leg in front of the other, crossing over. Feel the stretch in your inner thigh. The idea is to sweep the leg over the other. Don't swing!

REPEAT 2 sets of 8–12 reps.

BENEFITS: Tones and firms inner thighs.

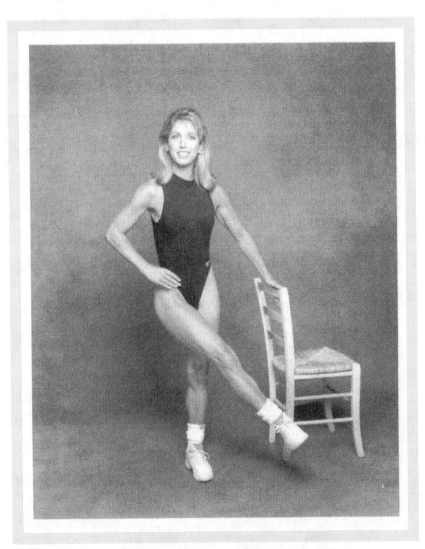

BOUNCE BACK WITH WEIGHTS

Here are four exercises that really work your muscles and will help you bounce back better than before!

Toning your body is just as important as trimming your after-baby weight. You know the old saying, "Use it or lose it"? Well, it's true!

When you reach the age of thirty-three, you start to lose muscle mass. That means you need to work about five minutes each day to achieve sculpted sexy arms and a nicely toned upper back and lifted chest. All you need is a pair of one- to five-pound dumbbells.

Remember, start slowly and increase your activity gradually.

1–6 weeks postpartum	=	5 reps
6–12 weeks postpartum	=	10 reps
3–4 months postpartum	=	15 reps
4 months and on	=	20 reps

Bounce Back Overhead Presses

Stand with your feet shoulder-width apart, abs tight, back straight, and knees slightly bent. Start with your hands at your shoulders, and exhale as you raise your hands over your head. Lower your arms to your shoulders and repeat.

REPEAT 2 sets of 8–12 reps. Rest 15 seconds between sets.

BENEFITS: Shoulders (deltoids), triceps.

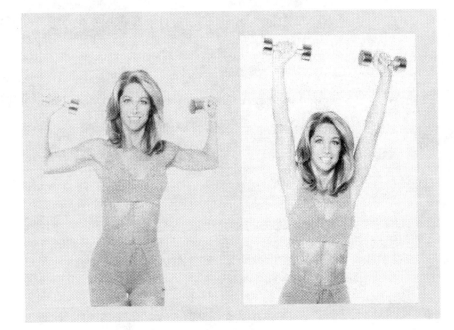

Bounce Back Tricep Toner

Stand with your feet apart, left foot in front of the right. Bend your knees slightly, and keep your abs tight. Rest the palm of your left hand on your left thigh. Holding the weight in your right hand, let your arm extend to the floor. Pull the weight up to your armpit, then lower it back to the starting position and repeat.

REPEAT 2 sets of 8–12 reps each per arm. Rest 15 seconds between sets.

BENEFITS: Upper back (latissimus dorsi, rhomboid), back of shoulders (posterior deltoid).

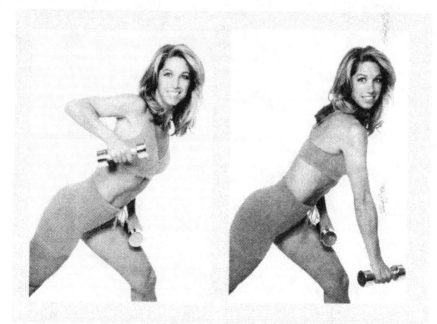

Bounce Back Shoulder Shape-up

Stand with your feet shoulder width apart, abs tight, back straight, and knees slightly bent.

Start with your hands at your side. With straight arms (don't lock elbows), lift the weights to the side slightly above shoulder level. Palms are down. Return to the starting position.

REPEAT 2 sets of 8–12 reps each. Rest 15 seconds between sets.

BENEFITS: Shoulders (medial deltoids).

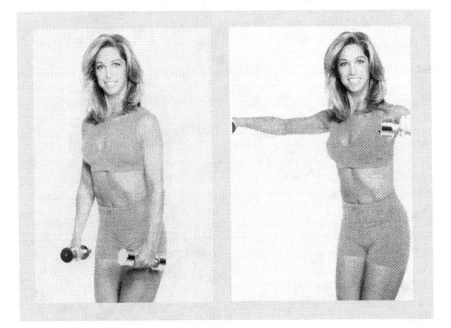

Bounce Back Chest Firmer

Lie on your back with your knees bent and your feet flat on the floor. Hold the weights in your hands with your arms extended straight out at shoulder level, above your chest with palms facing inward. Slowly lower your arms to your side, keeping them bent at the same angle throughout the movement. Slowly return your arms to the starting position by squeezing your chest as if to make cleavage and then repeating the movement.

REPEAT 2 sets of 8–12 reps each. Rest 15 seconds between sets.
BENEFITS: Chest (pectorals).

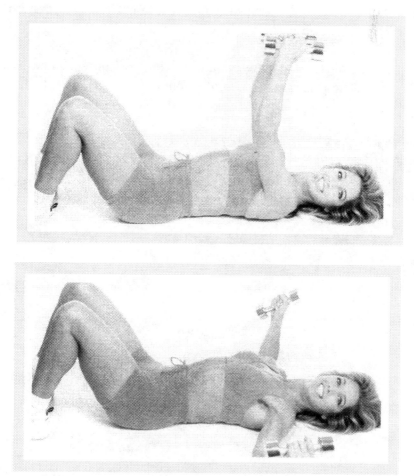

Stretching

■

OUR NEXT AREA of bouncing back to a better you is **stretching**. What are the benefits of stretching?

- **BETTER POSTURE**
- **BETTER BALANCE**
- **GRACE AND FLEXIBILITY**

As we age, flexibility does become more important, and ultimately stretching our bodies is a way to stay supple. Stretching will also help you in your daily routine with the baby . . . bending over the crib, keeping your back pliable, reeducating your upper back muscles to improve posture. Stretching also releases tension and makes you feel loose and relaxed.

Get into the habit of a five-minute stretching routine every day. This should be done after you exercise, when your muscles are nice and warm.

AFTER-BABY TIPS ON STRETCHING

1. Don't lock your joints—especially your knees.
2. Don't bounce. Hold each stretch for 1–20 seconds. Otherwise you could tear muscle fibers.
3. Do take it slowly, and *don't* overstretch.

Full Body Stretch

·

This is a super stretch for your whole body, especially your arms, shoulders, and spine; you can do this one either sitting or standing, and it's a great way to rejuvenate after sitting at your desk for long periods of time.

1. Lift your arms above your head and make yourself as tall as you can.
2. Make sure you breathe while holding the stretch for 5–15 seconds.
3. Bring your arms down in front of you and relax.

Variation: Side stretch—slowly bend slightly to the left and then to the right.

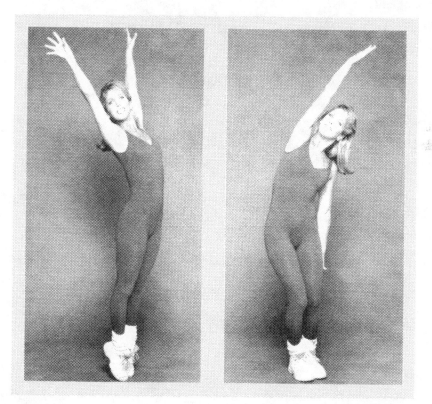

Lower Back

This lower back stretch is one of my favorites. It's easy to do, and it feels great! When performing this stretch, make sure you move smoothly; you don't want this to be a jerky movement.

1. Sit on the floor with your legs straight out in front of you.
2. Put your right foot on the outside of your left knee.
3. Place your left elbow on the outside of your right knee while reaching back with your right hand.
4. Look back over your right shoulder and feel the stretch in your lower back as you twist.
5. Hold stretch for 15–20 seconds, then repeat on the other side.

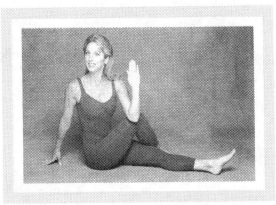

Hamstrings

.

I do this stretch all the time, whether I'm in bed, lying on the floor playing with the girls, or just watching television. It is especially useful if your lower back is bothering you. As with the rest of your stretches, be sure to breathe, relax, and never bounce!

1. Lie on your back on the floor, with your knees bent and your feet on the floor.
2. Raise your right leg and pull it toward your chest. You can use a towel to assist you.
3. Hold the stretch for 15–20 seconds.
4. Lower the leg and repeat the stretch with the left leg.

Variation: To feel stretch more in calf muscle, wrap towel around ball of foot.

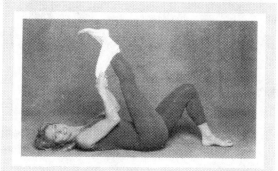

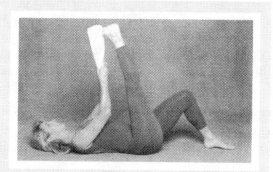

Quads

.

Your quadriceps are the four muscles in the front of your thighs. They are among the largest and strongest muscle groups in your body and are used in every activity. Jogging, biking, climbing, and even walking will be enhanced by having flexible thighs.

1. Lie on your side with your legs together.
2. Bend your right leg behind you and grasp the foot or the ankle.
3. Gently pull your foot toward your buttocks.
4. When you feel tension in the front of your thighs, hold the stretch 15–20 seconds.
5. Switch sides and repeat the movement with the left leg.

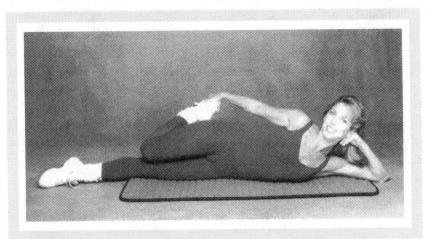

Afterword

*E*verybody always asks me if I am going to have a third child.

Don't you want to try for a boy?

Well, I'm forty-one years old, and it isn't out of the question. I don't want to say it won't happen. In fact, I still might go for it!

Having a baby is the most miraculous experience life has to offer. Enjoy your baby now, because they sure grow up fast! You forget the dirty diapers, the spit-up on your best blouse, the nights of lost sleep, the days of feeling frustrated by a colicky baby. You will never forget the smell of your baby's head. The sweetness of their breath on your cheek. Their first real smile (not gas!). The look in their eyes when they gaze up at you while you are feeding them and they gradually learn to grab your finger. It's the greatest love you will ever feel.

I can't tell you how much joy my two daughters have brought me and Jeff—and continue to every day of our lives. We are a family. It seems only yesterday I was walking with Jeff, holding hands and planning for our future. Well, our future is here! And it is better than I could even have imagined.

Sure, nobody is perfect, and no family is without stress. I know that balancing your life is hard. As a mother, there are times when I feel overwhelmed. And you will probably feel the same. From the moment I wake up in the morning until I go to bed, the race is on. Between getting up, working out, getting the kids up and out the door to school, running errands, cleaning house, doing chores, work, spending time with the kids, and making dinner, it's hard sometimes to see what is most important. I just try to realize that on some days things aren't going to get done.

Having a happy family life requires balance. To make it work, you need to help each other, believe in each other, and support each other.

My greatest wish for you is to be a healthy mom and a happy mom. Your child will reflect your beauty and spirit.

It is your greatest gift to them.

Index

chicken:
    rosemary roasted, with crispy potatoes, 91
    salad with oranges, warm, 193
Chick-Fil-A, 130
childbirth:
    late, 124, 165
    premature, 18, 124
childbirth classes, 49, 120
chloasma, 70, 77
chocolate:
    craving for, 85
    in frozen mousse pie, 196
    shake, 42
chromium, 28
chutney, melon, grilled salmon with, 40
Clapp, James F., 18–19
cleaning products, safety guidelines for, 22
clothes, 72–75
    exercise and, 47–48, 64
    for postpartum period, 180–81
cobbler, old-fashioned fruit, 94
colostrum, 123
concealer, 70
conception, 19
confidence, 14
constipation, 86–87, 161
contractions, 124, 163
copper, 28
cottage cheese, 30
cramps, 19, 120, 121
    amniocentesis and, 77
    exercise and, 113
cravings, see food cravings
cream cheese, light, in frozen mousse pie, 196
creamy foods, craving for, 85
crunchy foods, craving for, 85
C-sections, 18, 124, 162, 169
    exercise after, 171

dairy products, 29, 33
dehydration, 20, 28, 61, 137, 163
delivery, see labor and delivery
Denise's daily dose, 86
Denise's guilt-free shakes, 42
Denise's meatloaf, 89
depression, postpartum, 172, 182
desserts, 187
    frozen mousse pie, 196
    old-fashioned fruit cobbler, 94
diabetes, 137
diarrhea, 137
diet drinks, 31
dinner, 35, 87, 133, 187, 192
doctors, questioning of, 18, 21–22, 61
Domino's, 129
drugs, 22, 165
due date, calculation of, 22

eating and nutrition:
    for breast-feeding, 175, 184, 187, 189–90
    in fast-food restaurants, 127–30
    in first trimester, 19–21, 24–43
    in postpartum shape-up, 184–96
    in restaurants, 127–30, 138–39
    safety concerns and, 22, 137
    in second trimester, 80–95
    in third trimester, 126–39
    tips for, 21
    vitamins and minerals and, 26–28
    see also meal plans; recipes; specific foods
eating for two, 94
eating habits, good, importance of, 24, 30
eating plan, foods to include in, 29
edema, 164
eggs, in food pyramid, 33
embryo, 19
endorphins, 159
energy:
    diet and, 32, 185–87
    exercise and, 159
    lack of, 42, 44, 48–49
    return of, 47, 72, 117–18, 119
epidurals, 165
episiotomy, 162
ESPN, 72, 73
evening primrose oil, 48
exercising, 13
    aerobic, see aerobics
    benefits of, 18–19, 49–50, 158, 161–62
    calorie requirements and, 20
    circulation, 76
    clothes for, 47–48
    conditions that restrict, 45–46
    endorphins and, 159
    in first trimester, 18, 19, 44–69
    with husbands or partners, 48–49
    isometric, 164
    kegels, 115, 162
    labor and delivery benefits of, 18–19, 161–62
    in post-baby shape-up, 170–73, 197–226
    questions about, 112–14, 161–64
    safety concerns and, 22, 44–47, 64, 158, 159–60
    in second trimester, 96–115
    skipping of, 11–12
    sports modifications and, 60–62
    stopping of, 162–63
    in third trimester, 140–64
    warning signs and, 46
    water, 62, 76, 158, 163
    weight training and, 64, 163, 198, 217–21
"expectant" ab exercise, 110
eye makeup, 63, 122

About the Author

At 5 feet 4 inches and 112 pounds, Denise Austin has been dubbed "America's favorite fitness expert." Born on February 13, 1957, Denise grew up in San Pedro, California. She started gymnastics at the age of twelve and earned an athletic scholarship to the University of Arizona. She transferred to California State University, Long Beach, where she earned her degree in 1979. She began teaching aerobic exercise classes in the Los Angeles area, earning her own local television program two years later. In 1983, Denise married Jeff Austin, a sports attorney and brother of tennis champ Tracy Austin. They moved to Washington, D.C., when Jeff accepted a job with a sports marketing firm.

From 1984–1988, Denise was the resident fitness expert on NBC's *Today* show. She also wrote a column for the *Washington Post* and received a prestigious award from the President's Council on Physical Fitness and Sports.

In 1987 Denise created her ESPN television show, *Getting Fit.* Today she is seen on Lifetime television's *Denise Austin's Daily Workout* and on her new show, *Denise Austin's Fit and Lite.* She spends four months a year taping her popular programs at the most beautiful resorts in the world, traveling with her family as often as possible. Her television show, which has aired for more than fourteen years, is rated #1 and is seen in eighty-two countries. She is also the fitness expert of PBS's weekly television show *HealthWeek.* Denise has her own "Ask Denise" column in *Healthy Living* magazine.

Denise has created more than twenty-five bestselling exercise videos, has her own line of activewear and workout equipment, and appears monthly on QVC. She can be seen motivating people on talk shows and is often used as a fitness expert for magazine articles. Her sensible, realistic, and enthusiastic approach to fitness (she works out only 30 minutes a day) and eating (she never skips a meal) has won fans throughout the United States, from whom she receives over 700 letters a week. Making a difference in the lives of people and her strong belief that she can inspire people to feel better about themselves are what gives Denise the energy to tackle challenges and achieve her success.

She was honored with the distinguished alumna award of 1997 by her alma mater and gave the commencement address to the graduates. She is an honorary board member of former Surgeon General, C. Everett Koop, M.D.'s, "Shape Up America." She was appointed by Governor George Allen of Virginia as chairman of the governor's Commission on Physical Fitness and Sports.

A dynamo of energy in a size 5, Denise Austin is a true motivator and has become a veritable fitness empire. But Denise believes her greatest achievement yet is being a mom to her two daughters, Kelly and Katie.

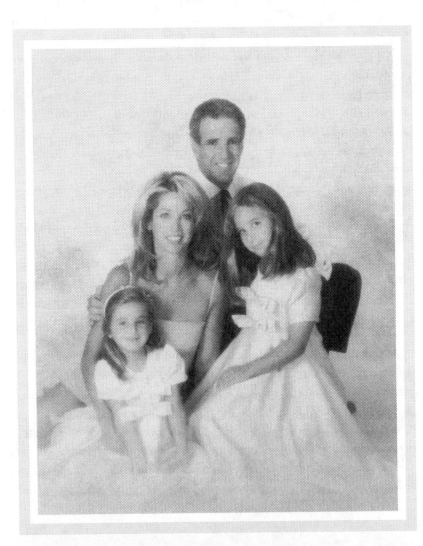

"Make The Best Time Of Your Life Even Better!"

BOUNCE BACK AFTER BABY Item #963 (45 minutes)
Designed to help women reclaim their waistline and keep up with the demands of a new baby. By using this program regularly, in addition to a healthy diet plan, women should begin to see results in as little as three weeks. Perfect for new Moms.

- A complete fat burning and firming program for tummy, hips, thighs, and buttocks.
- Includes a special energy building & relaxation segment.
- Special tips for women who've had a Cesarean section.
- Fun and easy to follow moves set to a great oldies soundtrack.

DENISE AUSTIN

Pregnancy Plus Workout

BONUS: A 20 Minute After Baby Shape Up

Star of ESPN's "Getting Fit With Denise Austin"

onforms with the guidelines of the American College of Obstetricians and Gynecologists"

NANCY PLUS Item #50 (60 minutes)
ned to keep women in shape during their entire nancy, this safe, easy-to-follow program con- to the guidelines set by the American College stetricians and Gynecologists.

proves overall energy level and stamina
elps relieve back pain and leg cramps
proves posture, circulation and digestion
cludes a 20-minute "After Baby Shape-Up" segment!

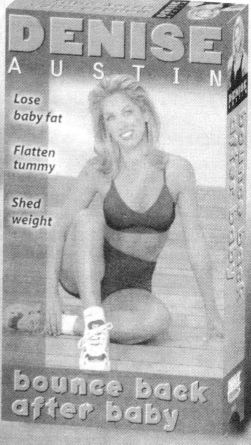

DENISE AUSTIN

Lose baby fat

Flatten tummy

Shed weight

bounce back after baby

PARADE VIDEO

Please consult your OB/GYN before beginning these exercise programs!

PPI Entertainment

Go With The Leader And Get Results!"

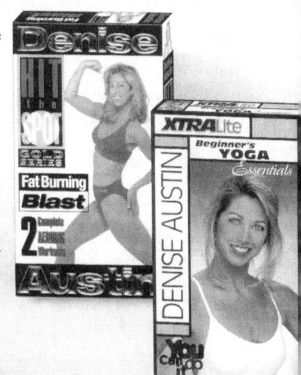